QUESTIONS AND ANSWERS FOR THE
DRCOG

SECOND EDITION

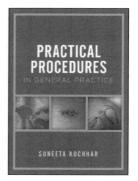

QUESTIONS AND ANSWERS FOR THE
DRCOG

SECOND EDITION

SUNEETA KOCHHAR

MBBS, MRCGP (2010), MRCS (2007), DRCOG, DFSRH

GP Principal in East Sussex

AND

PRABHA SINHA

MBBS, FRCOG, MRCPI

Consultant Obstetrician and Gynaecologist in East Sussex

Scion

© **Scion Publishing Limited, 2014**

ISBN 978 1 907904 19 6

Second edition first published 2014

First edition published 2011, reprinted 2011, 2012, 2013

A CIP catalogue record for this book is available from the British Library.

Scion Publishing Limited

The Old Hayloft, Vantage Business Park, Bloxham Road, Banbury OX16 9UX, UK

www.scionpublishing.com

Important Note from the Publisher

The information contained within this book was obtained by Scion Publishing Ltd from sources believed by us to be reliable. However, while every effort has been made to ensure its accuracy, no responsibility for loss or injury whatsoever occasioned to any person acting or refraining from action as a result of information contained herein can be accepted by the authors or publishers.

Readers are reminded that medicine is a constantly evolving science and while the authors and publishers have ensured that all dosages, applications and practices are based on current indications, there may be specific practices which differ between communities. You should always follow the guidelines laid down by the manufacturers of specific products and the relevant authorities in the country in which you are practising.

Although every effort has been made to ensure that all owners of copyright material have been acknowledged in this publication, we would be pleased to acknowledge in subsequent reprints or editions any omissions brought to our attention.

Registered names, trademarks, etc. used in this book, even when not marked as such, are not to be considered unprotected by law.

Typeset by Phoenix Photosetting, Chatham, Kent, UK

Printed in the UK

Contents

Preface

The DRCOG (Diploma of the Royal College of Obstetricians and Gynaecologists) is a knowledge-based certificate awarded following a written examination. The content is based on obstetrics and gynaecology relevant to general practice in the United Kingdom. The examination reflects common clinical scenarios encountered in general practice and includes sexual health and family planning. It does not represent a specialist qualification.

The Royal College of Obstetricians and Gynaecologists (RCOG) provide a curriculum and syllabus to aid revision for the examination. The syllabus includes modules on: Basic Clinical Skills, Basic Surgical Skills, Antenatal care, Management of Labour and Delivery, Postpartum Problems (The puerperium) including neonatal problems, Gynaecological Problems and Fertility Control (Contraception and termination of pregnancy).

The DRCOG examination is usually held twice a year, in April and October in a number of locations in the United Kingdom. The examination regulations state that candidates must hold full, limited or provisional registration with the General Medical Council. The examination may not be attempted more than 5 times. No training requirement is required to undertake the examination. As the question papers vary in difficulty the pass mark is variable; therefore there is no fixed pass rate. There is no negative marking.

The examination consists of a 3 hour written paper consisting of two 1½ hour papers. The first paper has 10 Extended Matching Questions (EMQs) each with 3 question items and 18 Single Best Answer (SBA) questions where a single answer is chosen from a list of five. It is recommended that two-thirds of the time for this paper is spent on the EMQs. Following a 15 minute break, the second paper is undertaken. The second paper consists of 40 five-part multiple choice questions (MCQs).

It is anticipated that the candidate may use this book for mock examination purposes therefore explanations are given at the end of each paper. The questions are based on common clinical scenarios and evidence-based explanations are given. The format is similar to the actual examination. It is intended that the candidate allows 3 hours to complete each exam paper, as recommended by the RCOG. Alternatively the book may be used to practice different question styles in separate sittings to aid revision. Furthermore this book may be helpful in preparing for the MRCGP Applied Knowledge Test and for medical finals.

Since the first edition a further practice examination has been added to the original three to aid revision. The original content has been reviewed and revised to reflect current guidance and the new examination paper has been written to complement the existing material.

Good luck!

Dr Suneeta Kochhar and Miss Prabha Sinha

About the authors

Suneeta Kochhar is GP Principal at Pebsham Surgery in Bexhill-on-Sea, in East Sussex. She completed the Membership of the Royal College of General Practitioners (MRCGP) in 2010 and completed the Membership of the Royal College of Surgeons (MRCS) examination in 2007. She also has the Diploma of the Royal College of Obstetricians and Gynaecologists (DRCOG) and the Diploma of the Faculty of Sexual and Reproductive Healthcare (DFSRH). She has published numerous educational articles.

Prabha Sinha is a Consultant Obstetrician and Gynaecologist at the Conquest Hospital in St Leonards-on-Sea, in East Sussex. She is also Honorary Consultant in Fetal Medicine at Guy's and St Thomas' Hospitals in London. She has Fellowship of the Royal College of Obstetricians and Gynaecologists (FRCOG) and Membership of the Royal College of Physicians of Ireland (MRCPI). She is involved in postgraduate education and assessment. She has examined for the DRCOG and currently examines for the Membership of the Royal College of Obstetricians and Gynaecologists (MRCOG) as well as the GMC exam for overseas doctors. She is also a teacher on MRCOG courses nationally and internationally.

DRCOG Syllabus

The Royal College of Obstetricians and Gynaecologists (RCOG) provide a curriculum and syllabus to aid revision for the examination. The syllabus refers to a level of knowledge appropriate to a General Practitioner in the United Kingdom. The syllabus may be updated in due course and it is advised that candidates refer to the RCOG website to check for the very latest information. The modules are listed and summarized below.

Module 1: Basic clinical skills

An understanding of symptomatology in patients presenting with gynaecological and obstetric problems as well as knowledge of sexually transmitted infections and family planning is expected. An understanding of pathophysiology and its clinical significance in addition to the risks and benefits of investigations and therapeutic interventions is expected. The syllabus places an emphasis on the medico-legal as well as ethical aspects of obstetrics and gynaecology. This includes the legal status of the unborn child, medical confidentiality and consent.

Module 2: Basic surgical skills

An understanding of commonly performed surgical procedures with an awareness of risks and benefits of therapeutic intervention is important. This encompasses an awareness of pre-operative investigations, pre- and post-operative care.

Module 3: Antenatal care

Knowledge related to peri-conceptual and antenatal care as well as the maternal complications of pregnancy is expected. This includes an understanding of psychiatric issues, domestic violence and cultural sensitivity. Furthermore, understanding how common medical disorders, antenatal screening and therapeutics impact on pregnancy is relevant. Moreover, the RCOG states that an understanding of the roles of other professionals underpins teamwork and effective communication skills.

Module 4: Management of labour and delivery

Knowledge and understanding that allows initial management of intrapartum problems in a hospital and in a community setting are required. Specifically, knowledge regarding obstetric emergencies, normal and abnormal labour, instrumental/Caesarean deliveries and obstetric anaesthesia, induction and augmentation of labour as well as assessment of fetal wellbeing is expected. Psychosocial aspects of obstetric care should be considered.

Module 5: Postpartum problems (the puerperium) including neonatal problems

Knowledge of postpartum problems and complications is expected. This includes an understanding of psychological disorders, therapeutics and management of neonatal problems which may include resuscitation.

Module 6: Gynaecological problems

This module encompasses knowledge and management skills related to urogynaecology, paediatric gynaecology, endocrine problems, pelvic pain, early pregnancy loss, investigation and management of male and female fertility problems, abnormal vaginal bleeding and sexually transmitted infections. Knowledge of malignant and premalignant conditions of the female genital tract, national screening programmes and palliative care is expected.

Module 7: Fertility control (contraception and termination of pregnancy)

Knowledge and understanding of reversible and irreversible contraceptive methods is expected, as well as termination of pregnancy. Medico-legal aspects related to abortion, consent and child protection are incorporated in this module. The RCOG state that whilst there may be conscientious objection to certain aspects of sexual and reproductive health, knowledge and understanding is expected.

Reference

Examination Committee (2007) *DRCOG Syllabus*. Royal College of Obstetricians and Gynaecologists

Abbreviations

AEDs	Anti-epileptic drugs
AFP	alpha-fetoprotein
APH	Antepartum haemorrhage
BMI	Body mass index
BNF	British National Formulary
BV	Bacterial vaginosis
CAH	Congenital adrenal hyperplasia
CMV	Cytomegalovirus
CS	Caesarean section
CSM	Committee on Safety of Medicines
CT	Computed tomography
CTG	Cardiotocography
CVS	Chorionic villus sampling
DDH	Developmental dysplasia of the hip
DMPA	Depot medroxyprogesterone acetate
DNA	Deoxyribonucleic acid
DVT	Deep vein thrombosis
ECG	Electrocardiogram
ELISA	Enzyme-linked immunosorbent assay
FSH	Follicle-stimulating hormone
GBS	Group B streptococcus
GnRH	Gonadotrophin-releasing hormone
HAART	Highly active anti-retroviral therapy
Hb	Haemoglobin
hCG	Human chorionic gonadotrophin
HIV	Human immunodeficiency virus
HNPCC	Hereditary non-polyposis colorectal cancer
HPV	Human papilloma virus
HRT	Hormone replacement therapy
HSV	Herpes simplex virus
IUD	Intrauterine device
IUGR	Intrauterine growth restriction
LARC	Long-acting reversible contraception
LDH	Lactate dehydrogenase
LFT	Liver function test
LH	Luteinising hormone

MMR	Measles, mumps, rubella (vaccine)
MRI	Magnetic resonance imaging
NAATs	Nucleic acid amplification tests
NICE	National Institute for Health and Care Excellence
NOMAC	Nomegestrol acetate
OHSS	Ovarian hyperstimulation syndrome
PAPP-A	Pregnancy-associated plasma protein A
PE	Pulmonary embolism
PID	Pelvic inflammatory disease
PCR	Polymerase chain reaction
PCOS	Polycystic ovary syndrome
PKU	Phenylketonuria
PM	Premenstrual syndrome
PPH	Postpartum haemorrhage
PROM	Pre-labour rupture of membranes
PUPPP	Pruritic urticated papules and plaques of pregnancy
RCOG	Royal College of Obstetricians and Gynaecologists
RNA	Ribonucleic acid
SGA	Small-for-gestational-age
SSRIs	Selective serotonin reuptake inhibitors
UAE	Uterine artery embolisation
UI	Urinary incontinence
UTI	Urinary tract infection
VIN	Vulval intraepithelial neoplasia
VZV	Varicella zoster virus
WHO	World Health Organization

Exam paper 1

Extended matching questions

Options for questions 1–3

A	Early pregnancy	F	Incomplete miscarriage
B	Threatened miscarriage	G	Complete miscarriage
C	Missed miscarriage	H	Menorrhagia
D	Molar pregnancy	I	Ectopic pregnancy
E	Retained products of conception	J	Pregnancy of unknown location

Instructions: for each of the patients described below, choose the **single** most appropriate diagnosis from the list above. Each option may be used once, more than once or not at all.

Question 1	A 26 year old woman self-referred to the Accident & Emergency department feeling faint. She had severe 'period-like pain' and a 15 day history of vaginal spotting. Her urine pregnancy test was positive.
Question 2	A 33 year old P1+0 woman was admitted by her GP with a heavy delayed period. On pelvic examination there were clots in the vagina and the cervical os was open. Her urine pregnancy test was positive.
Question 3	A 16 year old was admitted with abdominal pain and vaginal bleeding with passage of multiple fleshy vesicles. Her urine pregnancy test was positive and the serum beta hCG was 1 000 000 IU/ml

Options for questions 4–6

A	Empty uterus	F	Yolk sac only
B	Empty gestational sac	G	Fetal pole visible
C	Collapsed gestational sac	H	Yolk sac and fetal pole
D	Fluid in the pouch of Douglas	I	Molar appearance
E	Subchorionic haemorrhage	J	Endometrial thickness of 50mm

Instructions: for each of the patients described below, choose the **single** most appropriate diagnosis from the list above. Each option may be used once, more than once or not at all.

Question 4	A 22 year old woman had her first ultrasound scan in the early pregnancy unit. She is confident that her last menstrual period was 8 weeks ago. She was offered another scan in 2 weeks.
Question 5	A 32 year old woman who is 10 weeks pregnant was referred by her GP with a 10 day history of vaginal spotting. Her previous scan demonstrated a viable pregnancy.
Question 6	A 21 year old smoker with a history of a previous laparoscopy for an ectopic pregnancy was scanned in the early pregnancy unit for worsening pelvic pain and serum beta hCG of 5000 IU/ml. She had an empty uterus on transvaginal ultrasound.

Options for questions 7–9

A	Vaginal hysterectomy	F	Transcervical resection of endometrium
B	Subtotal hysterectomy	G	Manchester repair
C	Mirena coil	H	Depo-Provera
D	Endometrial curettage	I	Tranexamic acid
E	Microwave endometrial ablation	J	Uterine artery embolisation

Instructions: for each of the patients described below, choose the **single** most appropriate management option from the list above. Each option may be used once, more than once or not at all.

Question 7	A 45 year old multiparous Afro-Caribbean woman, with a BMI of 50, was referred to outpatients by her GP with worsening menorrhagia. She had an incidental finding of multiple fibroids when she was investigated for abdominal pain 10 years ago.
Question 8	A 49 year old woman attended the gynaecology outpatient clinic with worsening menorrhagia. She had the Mirena intrauterine system inserted 2 years ago which did not help her symptoms. She has a previous history of pulmonary embolism. Her previous ultrasound scan demonstrates a slightly bulky uterus.
Question 9	A 43 year old multiparous woman was referred by her GP with a dragging sensation and a feeling of fullness in the vagina. She also presented with worsening vaginal discharge and nearly continuous bleeding for six months. Her symptoms were adversely affecting her personal and professional life.

Options for questions 10–12

A	Chlamydia screening	F	Pelvic ultrasound
B	Partner semen analysis	G	Thyroid profile
C	Rubella immunity	H	Glucose tolerance test
D	Serum progesterone	I	Hysteroscopy
E	Serum oestrogen	J	Laparoscopy and dye test

Instructions: for each of the patients described below, choose the **single** most appropriate investigation from the list above. Each option may be used once, more than once or not at all.

Question 10	A 30 year old woman attended the gynaecology outpatient clinic with severe right-sided dyspareunia. She has been trying to conceive for 2 years. A recent infection screen was negative.
Question 11	A 28 year old woman has been trying to conceive for 2 years. She had a spontaneous conception and a Caesarean section four years ago. She had a perforated appendix 2 years ago.
Question 12	A 27 year old woman has been trying to conceive for 18 months. She has a five year old son from a previous relationship.

Options for questions 13–15

A	Urgent ultrasonography	F	Speculum examination
B	Abdominal and pelvic X-rays	G	Urgent laparoscopy
C	Pelvic examination	H	Laparotomy
D	Reassurance in the first instance	I	CT scan
E	MRI scan	J	Speculum examination followed by urgent ultrasonography

Instructions: for each of the patients described below, choose the **single** most appropriate investigation from the list above. Each option may be used once, more than once or not at all.

Question 13	A 26 year old woman complains of a 'lost' intrauterine contraceptive device. She does not give a history of spontaneous expulsion. Ultrasound examination does not identify the device.
Question 14	A 32 year old woman had an intrauterine device inserted 3 years ago. She cannot feel the threads from the device and is complaining of mild abdominal pain.
Question 15	A multiparous obese woman had an intrauterine contraceptive device inserted 1 month ago. She is unable to feel its threads.

Options for questions 16–18

A	Progesterone-only emergency contraception	F	Combined oral contraceptive
B	Intrauterine contraceptive device	G	Oestrogen patches
C	Cyproterone acetate	H	Progesterone-only implant
D	Vaginal ring	I	Depo-Provera
E	High dose oestrogen orally	J	Yasmin

Instructions: for each of the patients described below, choose the **single** most appropriate contraceptive from the list above. Each option may be used once, more than once or not at all.

Question 16	A 20 year woman presents to the Accident and Emergency department asking for the most effective emergency contraception for unprotected sexual intercourse 4 days ago.
Question 17	A 15 year old student visits her GP after unprotected intercourse yesterday.
Question 18	A 21 year old woman who does not like taking tablets and is not keen on long-acting reversible contraceptives wishes to discuss possible contraceptive options.

Options for questions 19–21

A	High vaginal swab (anterior wall)	F	Endocervical and urethral swabs
B	High vaginal swab (lateral wall)	G	Endocervical swab and nucleic acid amplification tests (NAATs)
C	Endocervical swab and culture	H	Enzyme-linked immunosorbent assay
D	High vaginal swab and saline wet microscopy	I	Polymerase chain reaction test
E	High vaginal swab and microscopy	J	Rectal and urethral swabs

Instructions: for each scenario below, choose the **single** most appropriate first-line investigation to diagnose the following conditions. Each option may be used once, more than once or not at all.

Question 19	*Trichomonas vaginalis* in women.
Question 20	*Chlamydia trachomatis* in a woman who requires an internal examination.
Question 21	Gonorrhoea in a woman who requires an internal examination.

Options for questions 22–24

A	Reassurance	F	Abdominal and pelvic X-rays
B	Transvaginal ultrasound at 28 weeks	G	CT scan
C	Transvaginal ultrasound at 36 weeks	H	MRI scan
D	Doppler ultrasonography	I	Angiogram
E	Admit to hospital	J	Cardiotocography at 37 weeks

Instructions: for each patient below, choose the **single** most appropriate first-line investigation. Each option may be used once, more than once or not at all.

Question 22	A 26 year old woman in her second pregnancy had her routine anomaly scan at 20 weeks. She was found to have a low-lying placenta that did not reach the cervical os.
Question 23	A 35 year old woman, with a history of three previous Caesarean sections, is 16 weeks pregnant. She is found to have an anterior, low-lying placenta on ultrasound scan.
Question 24	A 30 year old woman is found to have placenta praevia minor on her first trimester scan at 13 weeks. This is her first pregnancy.

Options for questions 25–27

A	Use condoms for 14 days	F	Take the missed pill as soon as possible and then continue taking it, abstain from sex or use barrier contraception until pills have been taken for 7 days in a row
B	No need for barrier contraception, consider emergency contraception	G	Do not use the combined oral contraceptive pill containing 20 micrograms of ethinyloestradiol.
C	Take the missed pill as soon as possible and then continue taking it	H	Omit the pill-free interval
D	Take the missed pill as soon as possible, use condoms for the next 7 days and consider emergency contraception.	I	Take the missed pill as soon as possible and then continue taking it, abstain from sex or use barrier contraception for the rest of the month
E	Offer immediate pregnancy testing	J	Switch to the progesterone-only pill

Instructions: for each scenario below, choose the **single** most appropriate contraceptive option from the list above. Each option may be used once, more than once or not at all.

Question 25	A 26 year old woman misses one combined oral contraceptive pill containing 20 mcg of ethinyloestradiol.
Question 26	A 35 year old woman misses two combined oral contraceptive pills containing 20 mcg of ethinyloestradiol in week one and has unprotected sexual intercourse.
Question 27	A 28 old woman misses two combined oral contraceptive pills containing 30 mcg of ethinyloestradiol during days 8–14 of her cycle.

Options for questions 28–30

A	Episiotomy	F	Forceps delivery
B	Wait and watch	G	Caesarean section
C	Assessment and review every 15 minutes	H	Offer amniotomy
D	Start oxytocin	I	Electronic fetal monitoring
E	Intermittent auscultation	J	Ventouse delivery

Instructions: for each scenario below, choose the **single** most appropriate option from the list above. Each option may be used once, more than once or not at all.

Question 28	A nulliparous woman has been in the active second stage of labour for 1 hour. On vaginal examination her membranes are intact.
Question 29	A multiparous woman has been in the active second stage of labour for 1 hour. Fetal monitoring is normal.
Question 30	A 28 year old woman in her second pregnancy is admitted to the labour ward. She presents at 40 weeks with contractions and there is meconium-stained liquor.

Single best answer questions

31 Which one of the following statements is **true**?

  A   Most cervical cancers are adenocarcinomas.

  B   Smoking cessation initially increases the risk of cervical cancer.

  C   The combined oral contraceptive pill increases the risk of cervical cancer.

  D   An Ayre spatula is used to sample the ectocervix for cervical screening.

  E   Gardasil vaccine for HPV (human papilloma virus) is recommended as part of the national immunisation campaign.

32 Concerning endometriosis, which one of the following options is **false**?

  A   Endometriosis is associated with pelvic pain.

  B   Subfertility is related to endometriosis.

  C   Endometriosis may cause haemoptysis.

  D   Treatment for endometriosis may involve the use of gonadotrophin-releasing hormone agonists.

  E   Symptoms of endometriosis worsen during pregnancy.

33 Regarding the progestogen-only intrauterine system Mirena, which one of the following statements is **false**?

  A   Mirena is licensed for the prevention of endometrial hyperplasia during oestrogen replacement therapy.

  B   Mirena is licensed for the treatment of menorrhagia.

  C   There is a rapid return to fertility on removal of the Mirena.

  D   Postpartum insertion should be delayed until 4 weeks.

  E   Mirena is effective for 4 years when used in conjunction with oestrogen replacement therapy.

34 Regarding hormone replacement therapy, which one of the following statements is **false**?

A   Continuous combined preparations are not suitable for use in the perimenopause.

B   Clonidine may be used to reduce vasomotor symptoms in women.

C   Hormone replacement therapy may be used as contraception.

D   A 49 year old women may be fertile for up to 2 years after her last menstrual period.

E   In women with a uterus, the addition of a cyclical progestogen reduces the risk of endometrial cancer.

35 Regarding management of urinary incontinence (UI), which one of the following statements is **true**?

A   Supervised pelvic floor muscle training for at least 2 months should be offered to women with stress or mixed UI.

B   Bladder training lasting for a minimum of 4 weeks should be offered to women with UI.

C   If bladder training is ineffective, extended release oxybutynin may be offered.

D   Pelvic floor muscle training should consist of at least eight contractions, three times a day.

E   Routine referral is indicated in women ≥40 years with recurrent urinary tract infections associated with haematuria.

36 Which one of the following is **not** a risk factor for cord prolapse?

A   Multiparity.

B   Artificial rupture of membranes.

C   Breech presentation.

D   Low lying placenta.

E   Oligohydramnios.

37 Which one of the following statements regarding obstetric cholestasis is **true**?

A Obstetric cholestasis affects 10% of women of Indian–Asian or Pakistani–Asian origin.

B It is associated with a typically very itchy rash.

C Postnatal resolution of liver function tests should be confirmed after 10 days.

D Bilirubin is frequently elevated.

E Pre-eclampsia does not affect liver function tests.

38 Which one of the following is **not** associated with shoulder dystocia?

A Decreased risk of postpartum haemorrhage.

B Diabetes.

C Prolonged second stage of labour.

D Perineal tears.

E Induction of labour.

39 Which one of the following statements concerning prenatal tests is **true**?

A Chorionic villus sampling is usually performed between 8 and 11 weeks of gestation.

B Chorionic villus sampling can be performed using a percutaneous transabdominal or transcervical approach.

C There is an approximately 2% risk of miscarriage associated with amniocentesis.

D Chorionic villus sampling can be used to screen for neural tube defects.

E Amniocentesis is used as a screening test.

40 Regarding screening for Down syndrome, which one of the following statements is **true**?

A   Diagnostic testing may be offered to a woman as a result of 1st trimester screening if the risk is greater than 1 in 300.

B   The combined test includes alpha-fetoprotein levels.

C   The combined test is performed at 15 weeks of gestation.

D   The combined test includes the nuchal translucency scan, human chorionic gonadotrophin and pregnancy-associated plasma protein A.

E   The integrated test does not include pregnancy-associated plasma protein A.

41 Which one of the following risks is **not** increased with Caesarean section?

A   Ureteric injury.

B   Venous thromboembolism.

C   Neonatal respiratory morbidity.

D   Uterovaginal prolapse.

E   Placenta praevia.

42 Which one of the following risks is **not** associated with diabetes during pregnancy?

A   Neonatal hyperglycaemia.

B   Pre-eclampsia.

C   Preterm labour.

D   Stillbirth.

E   Congenital malformations.

43 Which one of the following statements concerning heavy menstrual bleeding is **true**?

A   A biopsy is indicated for women ≥40 years if treatment is ineffective.

B   The levonorgestrel-releasing intrauterine system is a first-line treatment for menorrhagia.

C   Tranexamic acid is a hormonal treatment.

D   Norethisterone may be used at the beginning of the menstrual cycle.

E   Thyroid function tests should be performed.

44 Which one of the following statements is **false**?

A   Fluoxetine is the selective serotonin reuptake inhibitor with the lowest known risk during pregnancy.

B   Fluoxetine is found in breast milk at relatively high levels.

C   Paroxetine taken in the first trimester may be linked with fetal cardiac defects.

D   Selective serotonin reuptake inhibitors may be associated with an increased risk of persistent neonatal pulmonary hypertension if taken in the first trimester.

E   Women needing inpatient care for a mental disorder within 12 months of childbirth should be admitted to a specialist mother and baby unit.

45 Regarding consent issues, which one of the following statements is **false**?

A   All people ≥18 years are presumed to have capacity to consent, unless there is evidence to suggest otherwise.

B   Once an individual is 18 years old, no one can give consent on their behalf.

C   A competent person is able to understand and retain information relevant to their decision about their care.

D The Fraser guidelines involve trying to establish capacity.

E Contraceptives may be given to a patient aged under 16 years if she is likely to have sexual intercourse with or without contraceptive treatment.

46 Regarding emergency contraception, which one of the following statements is **true**?

A According to the manufacturer, levonorgestrel is effective if taken within 120 hours of unprotected sexual intercourse.

B According to the manufacturer, ulipristal is effective if taken within 120 hours of unprotected sexual intercourse.

C Levonorgestrel is more effective than the insertion of an intrauterine device.

D Barrier contraception does not need to be used following emergency hormonal contraception.

E A copper intrauterine contraceptive device can be inserted up to 72 hours after unprotected sexual intercourse.

47 Which one of the following statements is **false**?

A There is no limit on gestational age when considering termination of pregnancy if there is a risk to the mother's life.

B Anti-D immunoglobin should be given to non-sensitised Rhesus-negative women following termination of pregnancy.

C If a fetus is likely to be born with severe physical or mental abnormalities, an abortion may be performed at up to 24 weeks.

D If the continuance of pregnancy would involve risk to the mother's physical or mental health, an abortion may be performed at up to 24 weeks.

E If the continuance of pregnancy would involve risk to the physical or mental health of any existing child(ren), an abortion may be performed at up to 24 weeks.

48 Which one of the following statements is **true**?

A   Hypothyroidism occurs in approximately 10% of pregnant women.

B   Hypothyroidism in pregnancy is treated with a smaller dose of thyroxine when compared to the non-pregnant state.

C   Postpartum thyroiditis usually presents with pain.

D   Those with postpartum thyroiditis usually test negative for thyroid peroxidise antibodies.

E   During pregnancy there is an increase in thyroxine-binding globulin.

Multiple choice questions

For each of these multiple choice questions, you must indicate which of the statements are true and which are false.

49 Concerning cervical screening

A Women between the ages of 20 and 64 are eligible for cervical screening in England.

B Cervical screening is recommended every 3 years.

C In women who have never been sexually active, cervical screening is not recommended.

D Human papilloma viruses 16 and 18 are associated with cervical cancer.

E Smoking cessation reduces the risk of cervical cancer.

50 Concerning HIV and pregnancy

A Pregnancy accelerates HIV progression.

B Chorioamnionitis increases the risk of perinatal transmission.

C Preterm delivery decreases the risk of perinatal transmission.

D There is universal antenatal screening for HIV in the UK.

E Mother-to-child transmission may be reduced to 2%.

51 Galactorrhoea may be caused by the following

A Nipple stimulation.

B SSRIs.

C Acromegaly.

D Combined oral contraceptive pill.

E Phenothiazines.

52 Concerning ectopic pregnancy

A   It is associated with endometriosis.

B   It is associated with salpingitis.

C   It may present with shoulder tip pain.

D   It may be managed expectantly.

E   It may be managed laparoscopically.

53 Fibroids

A   Are more common in women who delay pregnancy.

B   Are less common in African women.

C   May present with subfertility.

D   May be associated with postpartum haemorrhage.

E   Are less likely to degenerate during pregnancy.

54 Concerning pelvic inflammatory disease (PID)

A   PID may cause perihepatic adhesions.

B   PID is associated with *Chlamydia trachomatis.*

C   PID always presents with cervical excitation.

D   PID may cause subfertility.

E   PID should prompt sexual health screening.

55 Concerning epilepsy and contraception

A   Periconceptual folic acid supplementation is recommended.

B   There is no risk of failure when carbamazepine is used with the combined oral contraceptive pill.

C   In women taking liver enzyme-inducing drugs who wish to use the combined oral contraceptive pill, a regimen using at least 40 mcg of oestrogen is recommended.

D After a liver enzyme-inducing medication is stopped, additional contraceptive cover is not needed.

E There is no risk of failure when ethosuximide is used with the combined oral contraceptive pill.

56 Hyperemesis gravidarum:

A Occurs in 20% of pregnancies.

B Is associated with low birth weight.

C Is associated with multiple pregnancy.

D May be related to gestational trophoblastic disease.

E Is commonly associated with thyroid problems.

57 Concerning neonatal resuscitation

A The airway is opened with the head slightly flexed.

B The ratio of compressions to inflations is 5:1.

C Stimulation may be provided by drying the baby.

D An inflation breath is given if breathing is inadequate at 90 seconds.

E Meconium should be aspirated from the baby's nose and mouth while the head is on the perineum.

58 Pre-eclampsia:

A Occurs at the 18th week of gestation.

B Is associated with proteinuria.

C May cause cerebral haemorrhage.

D May cause jaundice.

E May result in pulmonary oedema.

59 The following are risk factors for venous thromboembolism in pregnancy:

   A Antithrombin deficiency.

   B BMI >25 kg/m^2.

   C Pre-eclampsia.

   D Prolonged labour.

   E Inflammatory bowel disease.

60 Concerning periconceptual care

   A 5 mg folic acid supplementation is recommended for most women.

   B No vitamin supplementation is recommended.

   C Weight loss prior to conception may be advisable.

   D High caffeine intake may be associated with miscarriage.

   E Immunity against German measles should be checked prior to conception.

61 Concerning chicken pox and pregnancy

   A Varicella zoster virus (VZV) is an RNA virus.

   B Chicken pox is infectious 24 hours before the rash appears.

   C VZV immunoglobulin antibody levels are screened antenatally.

   D If a pregnant women not immune to VZV has been exposed, immunoglobulin may be given up to 5 days after contact.

   E Fetal varicella syndrome may be associated with limb hypoplasia.

62 Regarding sterilisation

   A Female sterilisation has an increased failure rate postpartum.

   B The lifetime risk of failure for tubal occlusion is approximately 1 in 2000.

C A pregnancy test is performed before surgery for tubal occlusion.

D The failure rate for vasectomy is 1 in 2000.

E A man is considered sterile when he has produced three consecutive semen samples with no spermatazoa.

63 With regards to routine antenatal screening in the UK, the following are tested for:

A Group B streptococcus.

B Hepatitis C virus.

C Hepatitis B virus.

D Syphilis.

E Varicella zoster antibodies.

64 Combined oral contraceptives:

A May be used to treat dysmenorrhoea.

B Increase the number of functional ovarian cysts.

C Increase the risk of ovarian cancer.

D Emergency contraception is recommended if three or more combined oral contraceptive pills are missed.

E If vomiting occurs within 3 hours of taking the combined contraceptive pill another pill should be taken.

65 Regarding management of urinary incontinence (UI)

A Women with UI should be advised to modify their fluid intake.

B Sacral nerve stimulation is recommended for the treatment of UI.

C Mid-urethral tape procedures may be used for stress UI.

D Microscopic haematuria if aged ≥50 years necessitates a routine referral.

E A 2 week wait referral is indicated for visible haematuria.

66 Planned Caesarean section should be offered to women with:

A Human immunodeficiency virus.

B Twin pregnancy where the first twin is breech.

C Hepatitis C virus.

D Recurrent genital herpes at term.

E Hepatitis B virus.

67 The following medications may safely be taken during pregnancy:

A Folic acid.

B Oral hypoglycaemia agents except metformin.

C Angiotensin-II receptor antagonists.

D Statins.

E Aspirin.

68 Concerning risk factors for postpartum haemorrhage (PPH)

A Placenta praevia increases the risk of PPH.

B Obesity decreases the risk of PPH.

C Delivery by emergency Caesarean section decreases the risk of PPH.

D Operative vaginal delivery decreases the risk of PPH.

E Pre-eclampsia increases the risk of PPH.

69 Concerning neonatal jaundice

A 30% of term babies develop jaundice in the first week of life.

B 50% of preterm babies develop jaundice in the first week of life.

C Jaundice is prolonged if it occurs for more than 14 days in term babies.

D Jaundice is prolonged if it occurs for more than 14 days in preterm babies.

E Physiological jaundice occurs in the first 24 hours of life.

70 Concerning epidural anaesthesia

A Epidural opioids do not cause respiratory problems in the newborn.

B Epidurals are associated with a longer first stage of labour.

C Epidurals are associated with a longer second stage of labour.

D Epidurals are associated with an increased risk of instrumental vaginal delivery.

E Epidurals are associated with an increased risk of Caesarean section.

71 Obesity in pregnancy:

A Increases the risk of venous thromboembolism.

B Increases the risk of gestational diabetes.

C Reduces the risk of pre-eclampsia.

D Reduces the risk of postpartum haemorrhage.

E Increases the risk of antepartum haemorrhage.

72 Regarding gonorrhoea

A *Neisseria gonorrhoeae* is a Gram positive diplococcus.

B The usual incubation period for gonorrhoea is up to 3 weeks.

C It does not cause dysuria in men.

D It is associated with pelvic inflammatory disease.

E In women it commonly presents with vaginal discharge.

73 Down syndrome may be associated with the following:

A Hypertonia.

B Cataracts.

C Hypothyroidism.

D Chronic myeloid leukaemia.

E Duodenal atresia.

74 Regarding anaemia and pregnancy

A Anaemia in pregnancy is usually caused by an increase in plasma volume.

B Antenatal screening for anaemia is recommended at 24 weeks.

C Antenatal screening for anaemia is recommended at 28 weeks.

D Hb <11 g/dl at the booking visit confirms anaemia.

E Iron preparations are more effective when taken with food.

75 Concerning intrauterine growth restriction (IUGR)

A Oligohydramnios may be suggestive of IUGR.

B IUGR may be a feature of fetal alcohol syndrome.

C Chromosomal abnormality usually causes asymmetric IUGR.

D Pre-eclampsia usually causes symmetric IUGR.

E Toxoplasmosis infection does not cause IUGR.

76 Regarding parvovirus B19

A Parvovirus B19 may be transmitted through blood products.

B The incubation period is up to 10 days.

C The presence of a rash indicates high infectivity.

D Infection at 16 weeks of gestation may cause fetal hydrops.

E Parvovirus B19 may cause aplastic crisis.

77 Concerning group B streptococcus

A Prolonged rupture of membranes is a risk factor for group B streptococcus infection in the neonate.

B Intrapartum pyrexia is not a risk factor for group B streptococcus infection in the neonate.

C Prematurity is not a risk factor for group B streptococcus infection in the neonate.

D Routine antenatal screening for group B streptococcus is carried out in the UK.

E Penicillin G may be used for intrapartum prophylaxis.

78 Concerning the menopause

A During the menopause there is a decline in progesterone levels.

B During the menopause there is a decline in luteinising hormone levels.

C Measuring hormone levels is diagnostic.

D During the menopause there is an increase in follicle stimulating hormone levels.

E Women may present with dyspareunia.

79 Regarding molar pregnancy

A Complete moles are triploid.

B Partial moles do not contain fetal tissue.

C Multiple pregnancy is a risk factor for molar pregnancy.

D Hydatidiform moles do not present with vaginal bleeding.

E Women with molar pregnancy should be on a register.

80 Regarding fetal circulation

A   Blood is returned from the placenta by the umbilical artery to the inferior vena cava.

B   The foramen ovale shunts deoxygenated blood from the right to the left atrium.

C   Blood is diverted from the descending aorta into the pulmonary trunk through the ductus arteriosus.

D   Closure of the foramen ovale is brought about by pressure changes in the atria.

E   Fetal haemoglobin has an oxygen dissociation curve that is shifted to the right when compared with adult haemoglobin.

81 Concerning sickle cell disease and pregnancy

A   Sickle cell disease is an X-linked autosomal recessive condition.

B   Sickle cell disease in pregnancy may cause intrauterine growth restriction.

C   Sickle cell disease in pregnancy does not increase the risk of intrauterine death.

D   Symptoms of sickle cell disease are immediately apparent in the neonate.

E   Screening should ideally be preconceptual.

82 Concerning developmental dysplasia of the hip (DDH)

A   DDH is not associated with breech presentation.

B   There is an increased risk of DDH in males.

C   Ultrasound is used routinely as a screening tool in the UK.

D   The Barlow test involves applying forward pressure to the femoral heads to relocate a dislocation or subluxation.

E   The Barlow test attempts to displace the hip by applying backward pressure to the head of the femur.

83 Regarding prematurity

A According to the World Health Organization, prematurity is defined as being born before 36 weeks of gestation.

B Pre-eclampsia is not a risk factor for prematurity.

C Polyhydramnios is a risk factor for prematurity.

D Premature babies have an increased risk of hyperglycaemia.

E Premature babies may receive immunisations according to their chronological age.

84 Regarding human immunodeficiency virus (HIV)

A There is universal antenatal testing of HIV in the UK.

B Universal testing of HIV is not recommended in sexual health clinics.

C Testing usually involves an assay for HIV antibody and p24 antigen.

D HIV causes a seroconversion illness 3 months after infection.

E Point of care tests from a fingerprick or mouth swab have a high specificity.

85 Regarding hormone replacement therapy (HRT)

A HRT does not increase the risk of ovarian cancer.

B HRT is associated with an increased risk of breast cancer within 3 years.

C The additional risk of breast cancer associated with HRT declines within 10 years of stopping HRT.

D In women aged 50–59 years there are six additional cases of breast cancer per 1000 women using combined HRT for 5 years.

E In women aged 50–59 years there are 24 additional cases of breast cancer per 1000 women using combined HRT for 5 years.

86 Concerning vasectomy

A Vasectomy is less invasive as a procedure when compared with female sterilisation.

B The lifetime risk of failure for tubal occlusion in women is approximately 1 in 200.

C The failure rate for vasectomy is 1 in 200 after clearance has been given.

D A man is considered sterile post-vasectomy when he has produced three consecutive semen samples with no spermatozoa.

E Vasectomy increases the risk of testicular cancer.

87 Regarding lactational amenorrhoea

A Breastfeeding delays ovulation.

B In the developed world, breastfeeding is not recommended in HIV-positive mothers.

C The lactational amenorrhoea method is approximately 80% effective in providing contraception.

D The lactational amenorrhoea method is more effective if women are less than 6 months postpartum.

E The lactational amenorrhoea method is most effective if women are not fully breastfeeding.

88 The NuvaRing (combined vaginal ring):

A Is contraindicated in those with latex allergy.

B May remain *in situ* during tampon use.

C Is refrigerated prior to dispensing.

D Has a shelf life of 6 months after being dispensed.

E Requires fitting by a health care professional.

Answers and explanations for exam paper 1

1. Answer I Ectopic pregnancy

The symptoms of an ectopic pregnancy are initially the same as for a normal pregnancy and typically start at around the 6th week of pregnancy. The symptoms include a missed period, nausea, and breast tenderness. Ectopic pregnancy may be associated with unilateral abdominal pain which may be persistent and severe. It may develop acutely or may develop over several days. Vaginal bleeding associated with ectopic pregnancy may be lighter, darker or watery. Ectopic pregnancy may cause internal bleeding which may in turn cause diaphragmatic irritation and pain referred to the shoulder tip. More than 50% of women with ectopic pregnancy are asymptomatic. They may present with collapse due to haemodynamic compromise.

2. Answer F Incomplete miscarriage

A miscarriage is called 'incomplete' where there is bleeding and cervical dilatation, but tissue from the pregnancy still remains in the uterus. In 90% of cases incomplete miscarriage resolves without any intervention.

3. Answer D Molar pregnancy

This is the commonest type of trophoblastic benign disease. In the UK this occurs in 0.1% of pregnancies and is three times more common in Asian women. Molar pregnancies usually present with painless vaginal bleeding in the fourth to fifth month of pregnancy; however, diagnosis is confirmed much earlier due to the routine use of ultrasound. There may be passage of 'grape-like' vesicles with bleeding. Molar pregnancy may present with persistent nausea and vomiting, ovarian cysts and 'large for dates'.

Hydatidiform moles may be complete or partial and this is dependent on genetic and histopathological features. Complete moles are diploid and there is no evidence of fetal tissue. Partial moles usually have some evidence of an abnormal fetus or fetal tissue. They are triploid in origin with a maternal set of haploid genes and two paternal sets of haploid genes.

4. Answer F Yolk sac only

The next structure after the gestational sac to become visible to ultrasound is the yolk sac as the pregnancy advances. This is a round, sonolucent structure with a bright rim. The yolk sac first appears during the fifth week of pregnancy and grows to be no larger than 6 mm. Yolk sacs larger than 6 mm are usually indicative of an abnormal pregnancy. Failure to identify a yolk sac on transvaginal ultrasound, when the gestational sac has grown to 12 mm, is usually indicative of a failed pregnancy.

The yolk sac is situated on the ventral aspect of the embryo. It is lined by extra-embyronic endoderm, outside of which is a layer of extra-embryonic mesenchyme, derived from the mesoderm. During the 6th week, cardiac activity should be apparent when the fetal pole is 5 mm long.

5. Answer E Subchorionic haemorrhage

Subchorionic haemorrhage or haematoma is the most common sonographic abnormality in the presence of a live embryo. Vaginal bleeding affects 25% of all women during the first half of pregnancy and is a common reason for first trimester ultrasonography. Sonographic visualisation of a subchorionic haematoma is important in a symptomatic woman because those with a demonstrable haematoma have a worse prognosis than women without. However, small asymptomatic subchorionic haematomas do not worsen prognosis and often regress. Large haematomas, which strip at least 30–40% of placenta away from the endometrium, may enlarge further causing compression of the gestational sac. This may lead to premature rupture of membranes with subsequent spontaneous abortion.

6. Answer D Fluid in the pouch of Douglas

In patients presenting with symptoms of ruptured ectopic pregnancy, there may be significant free fluid in the peritoneal cavity and pouch of Douglas detected on transvaginal ultrasound.

7. Answer J Uterine artery embolisation

Uterine artery embolisation (UAE) is an alternative to hysterectomy for fibroids. It is minimally invasive and is tolerated in those with concomitant disease. The procedure involves occluding the uterine arteries, usually with polyvinyl alcohol beads, using a transfemoral approach (under local anaesthesia and light sedation). This impairs blood supply to the fibroids and causes shrinkage and necrosis over a few weeks. Patients are in hospital for 24–36 hours and are advised to rest for 1–2 weeks. UAE is usually performed by an interventional radiologist.

8. Answer E Microwave endometrial ablation

Historically hysterectomy was seen as the standard treatment for women with menorrhagia who had not responded to medical treatment. Minimally invasive procedures to destroy the endometrium are alternatives to hysterectomy. They include the use of lasers, radiofrequency waves, electrocautery, heated saline, or a heated balloon. Microwave endometrial ablation is one of these minimally invasive procedures. It involves inserting a microwave probe into the uterine cavity to heat the endometrium.

9. Answer A Vaginal hysterectomy

In this scenario vaginal hysterectomy is considered the most effective treatment and is preferable to total abdominal hysterectomy. Vaginal hysterectomy may be associated with an increased risk of vaginal vault prolapse.

10. Answer F Pelvic ultrasound

Pelvic ultrasound may be used to investigate women presenting with lower abdominal pain. In this scenario, pelvic ultrasound may be used to exclude an ectopic pregnancy or ovarian pathology. Infertility refers to the failure to conceive after regular unprotected intercourse for 2 years in the absence of known reproductive pathology. An assessment of ovulation may be made by taking a menstrual history and by measuring day 21 serum progesterone in a 28 day cycle as well as serum gonadotrophins. Lifestyle advice for couples wishing to conceive includes advising regular intercourse, smoking cessation, BMI <30, and reducing alcohol intake. Preconceptual care includes screening for rubella susceptibility, advising about folic acid use and cervical screening.

11. Answer J Laparoscopy and dye test

In this scenario, there is a previous history of Caesarean section and appendicitis with perforation. Adhesions may cause tubal infertility.

12. Answer B Partner semen analysis

In couples who have failed to conceive after regular unprotected intercourse for 2 years, the male partner should normally undergo semen analysis. Laboratories that perform semen analysis should undertake this according to recognised World Health Organization methodology.

13. Answer B Abdominal and pelvic X-rays

Uterine or cervical perforation, displacement and expulsion are risks associated with intrauterine devices. The intrauterine device threads may be 'lost' if a woman has not recognised a spontaneous expulsion, if the threads have retracted into the cervix or uterus, or if there is perforation. Expulsion is more likely in nulliparous women. Management includes speculum examination to locate the threads and assessment of the risk of pregnancy. If this is unsuccessful, ultrasonography is carried out in the first instance and then X-ray examination should be considered. If perforation and migration of the intrauterine device is suspected surgical intervention is required.

14. Answer J Speculum examination followed by urgent ultrasonography

If speculum examination to locate threads is unsuccessful, ultrasonography is performed.

15. Answer **D** Reassurance in the first instance

In this scenario it is likely that the threads have retracted into the cervix or uterus therefore reassurance in the first instance is important. A speculum examination should be performed.

16. Answer **B** Intrauterine contraceptive device

Levonorgestrel and ulipristal are emergency hormonal contraceptives that should be taken as soon as possible after unprotected sexual intercourse. Levonorgestrel is licensed for use up to 72 hours; however, it may be used after this with reduced effectiveness. Ulipristal may be used within 120 hours of unprotected sexual intercourse. Ulipristal is as effective as levonorgestrel in preventing pregnancy, but it has not been compared with insertion of an intrauterine device. Levonorgestrel is less effective than the insertion of an intrauterine device. A copper intrauterine contraceptive device can be inserted up to 120 hours after unprotected sexual intercourse and is the most effective method of emergency contraception.

17. Answer **A** Progesterone-only emergency contraception

Levonorgestrel is licensed for use up to 72 hours and ulipristal may be used within 120 hours of unprotected sexual intercourse. In this scenario emergency hormonal contraception has been sought within 24 hours of unprotected sexual intercourse, therefore efficacy is at its highest at 98%. The efficacy for emergency hormonal contraception is up to 58% at 49–72 hours and the efficacy is up to 85% at 25–48 hours. Emergency hormonal contraception is a better option than copper intrauterine contraceptive device insertion in a 15 year old.

18. Answer **D** Vaginal ring

NuvaRing is a combined vaginal ring licensed for contraceptive use. It is a latex-free, flexible ring that is inserted into the vagina by the patient for 3 weeks per cycle, after this there is a ring-free week (analogous to the combined oral contraceptive pill-free interval).

19. Answer **D** High vaginal swab and saline wet microscopy

Trichomonas vaginalis is a protozoan. It may present with vulval itching, dysuria, abdominal pain and an offensive smelling yellow frothy discharge in women. In women it is usually diagnosed by taking a vaginal swab for saline wet microscopy. The pH of vaginal secretions may be >4.5 but this is not a specific feature. Swab culture is more specific and sensitive than saline wet microscopy. In men, culture is more useful as saline wet microscopy is more likely to be negative. Polymerase chain reaction (PCR) tests are not widely used.

20. Answer **G** Endocervical swab and nucleic acid amplification tests (NAATs)

Chlamydia is caused by an intracellular Gram-negative bacteria and it may be asymptomatic. Women may present with vaginal discharge, lower abdominal pain, dyspareunia, intermenstrual or postcoital bleeding. Urethritis may be the presenting feature in men. Long-term complications include infertility. It is an infection which may co-exist with other sexually transmitted infections. Chlamydial infection may result in urethritis, arthritis and conjunctivitis (Reiter's syndrome). A urethral swab in a male may be used to diagnose *Chlamydia,* however, this has been superseded by NAATs on first void urine samples. NAATs are more sensitive and specific when compared with enzyme-linked immunosorbent assays. In women, a self-administered vaginal swab may be taken; however, if an internal examination is performed an endocervical swab is usually taken.

21. Answer **F** Endocervical and urethral swabs

Neisseria gonorrhoeae is a Gram-negative diplococcus that is transmitted by inoculation of infected secretions between mucous membranes. In men, urethral swabs may be taken as well as rectal and oropharyngeal swabs if appropriate. In women, endocervical and urethral swabs may be taken routinely if a speculum examination is carried out. Gonorrhoea may also be identified using NAATs on first void urine samples. Microscopy of Gram-stained genital specimens may allow immediate diagnosis of gonorrhoea.

22. Answer **C** Transvaginal ultrasound at 36 weeks

Placenta praevia refers to insertion of the placenta into the lower segment of the uterus. If the placenta overlies the cervical os this represents major placenta praevia. If placenta praevia is suspected on the routine anomaly scan, transvaginal ultrasound should be performed. A transvaginal ultrasound should be repeated at 36 weeks if there is asymptomatic minor placenta praevia. In major placenta praevia imaging should be carried out at 32 weeks.

23. Answer **D** Doppler ultrasonography

Doppler ultrasonography should be performed in women with placenta praevia who are at risk of placenta accreta. In this scenario there is an increased risk of placenta accreta due to a previous history of Caesarean sections.

24. Answer **A** Reassurance

In this situation reassurance is appropriate because placental migration occurs during the second and third trimesters as the lower uterine segment develops. In most of these cases there is a normally situated placenta at term. If placenta praevia is suspected on the routine anomaly scan, transvaginal ultrasound should be performed.

25. Answer C Take the missed pill as soon as possible and then continue taking it

If 1–2 pills are missed in a woman taking the combined oral contraceptive pill with 30–35 mcg of ethinyloestradiol, the next pill should be taken as soon as possible. No additional contraceptive cover is needed. If three or more pills are missed in a woman taking the combined oral contraceptive pill with 30–35 mcg of ethinyloestradiol, the next pill should be taken as soon as possible. Furthermore, additional contraceptive precautions are needed until pills have been taken for 7 days in a row. If pills are missed in the third week, the pill-free interval should be omitted. If there are missed pills in the first week, emergency contraception should be considered if sexual intercourse took place in week 1 or the pill-free interval.

If one pill is missed in a woman taking the combined oral contraceptive pill with 20 mcg of ethinyloestradiol, no additional contraceptive cover is required. However, if two or more pills are missed in a woman taking the combined oral contraceptive pill with 20 mcg of ethinyloestradiol, additional precautions are needed until pills have been taken for 7 days in a row.

26. Answer D Take the missed pill as soon as possible, use condoms for the next 7 days and consider emergency contraception

27. Answer C Take the missed pill as soon as possible and then continue taking it

28. Answer H Offer amniotomy

In this scenario there is inadequate progress after 1 hour during the active second stage of labour. Vaginal examination should be offered and amniotomy advised if the membranes are intact. In nulliparous women, delay in the active second stage of labour is diagnosed if it has lasted 2 hours.

29. Answer C Assessment and review every 15 minutes

In multiparous women, delay in the active second stage of labour is diagnosed if it has lasted 1 hour. If there is a diagnosis of delay in the second stage there should be an assessment and review every 15–30 minutes by an obstetrician. Oxytocin should not be started and instrumental or operative delivery should be considered.

30. Answer I Electronic fetal monitoring

Continuous electronic fetal monitoring is recommended if there is significant meconium-stained liquor. Fetal blood sampling should be considered if there is concern about fetal distress.

31. Answer C

Smoking cessation is associated with a reduction in cervical cancer. The majority of cervical cancers are squamous carcinomas. The combined oral contraceptive pill decreases the risk of ovarian and endometrial cancer. There is an increased risk of cervical cancer with long-term oral contraceptive use. A brush rather than a spatula is used to sample the ectocervix for liquid-based cytology. There are two types of HPV vaccine currently available, Gardasil and Cervarix; the latter was chosen for the national immunisation programme. It is recommended that it is first given to girls at 12–13 years of age. (*NICE*, 2003; *Cervical cancer – cervical screening (review)*: *guidance*: TA69.)

32. Answer E

Endometriosis is a condition in which hormonally responsive endometrial tissue is found outside the uterus. Endometriosis is therefore generally confined to women in their reproductive years. Women may report dyspareunia; this is more likely to be a feature of severe disease. Moreover this may be associated with an immobile fixed retroverted uterus. Extra-abdominal manifestations include cyclical haemoptysis. Symptoms usually improve during pregnancy and after the menopause. Gonadotrophin-releasing hormone agonists can be used to significantly reduce oestradiol levels; therefore this treatment is very effective in resolution of active disease and pain reduction.

33. Answer D

The progestogen-only intrauterine system Mirena prevents endometrial proliferation, thickens cervical mucus and may cause suppression of ovulation. Postpartum insertion should be delayed until 6 weeks after delivery.

34. Answer C

Continuous combined preparations are not suitable for use in the perimenopause as women who use continuous preparations in this period are prone to irregular bleeding. Hormone replacement therapy does not provide contraceptive cover. A woman is considered fertile for 2 years after her last menstrual period if she is <50 years. A woman is considered fertile for 1 year after her last menstrual period if she is >50 years.

35. Answer D

A trial of supervised pelvic floor muscle training of at least 3 months' duration should be offered to women with stress or mixed UI. Bladder training lasting for a minimum of 6 weeks should be offered as first-line treatment to women with urge or mixed UI. Immediate release oxybutynin should be offered to women with an overactive bladder if bladder training has been ineffective. If immediate release oxybutynin is not well tolerated, solifenacin, tolterodine or extended release oxybutynin may be considered. An urgent referral is indicated in women ≥40 years with recurrent urinary tract infections associated with haematuria. (*NICE*, 2006; *Urinary incontinence*: CG40.)

36. Answer E

Risk factors for cord prolapse include multiparity, artificial rupture of membranes, low birth weight, prematurity, fetal congenital anomalies, breech presentation, polyhydramnios and abnormal placentation (*RCOG*, 2008; *Green-top Guideline 50: Umbilical cord prolapse*).

37. Answer C

Obstetric cholestasis affects up to 1.5% of women of Indian–Asian or Pakistani–Asian origin. It is characterised by intense pruritus without a skin rash, especially at night, and it is associated with abnormal liver function tests, both of which resolve after delivery. Obstetric cholestasis may be linked to prematurity and intrauterine death. Bilirubin is not commonly raised and most women will have increased levels of one or more of the liver function tests. Acute fatty liver of pregnancy and pre-eclampsia should be considered in the differential diagnosis. (*RCOG*, 2006; *Green-top Guideline 43: Obstetric cholestasis.*)

38. Answer A

Shoulder dystocia is associated with perinatal mortality and morbidity. There is an increased risk of postpartum haemorrhage and fourth-degree perineal tears with shoulder dystocia. Previous shoulder dystocia, prolonged first and second stages of labour, macrosomia, diabetes, induction of labour, maternal BMI >30 kg/m^2 are associated with shoulder dystocia. (*RCOG*, 2005; *Green-top Guideline 42: Shoulder dystocia.*)

39. Answer B

Most amniocentesis tests are performed from 15 weeks of completed gestation and chorionic villus sampling is usually performed between 10 and 13 weeks of gestation. Chorionic villus sampling can be performed using a percutaneous transabdominal or transcervical approach. There is an approximately 1% risk of miscarriage associated with amniocentesis. Chorionic villus sampling and amniocentesis are not used as screening tests.

40. Answer D

From 11 to 13^{+6} weeks of gestation the combined test may be performed. The combined test consists of the nuchal translucency scan, human chorionic gonadotrophin (hCG) and pregnancy-associated plasma protein A (PAPP-A). The quadruple test may be carried out from 15 to 20 weeks. This includes hCG, alpha-fetoprotein, unconjugated oestriol and inhibin A. From 11 to 13^{+6} weeks and 15–20 weeks, the integrated test includes the nuchal translucency scan, hCG, PAPP-A, alpha-fetoprotein, unconjugated oestriol, and inhibin A. Diagnostic testing may be offered to a woman as a result of 1st trimester screening if the risk is greater than 1 in 150.

41. Answer D

The following risks are increased with Caesarean section: bladder and ureteric injury, hysterectomy, venous thromboembolism, length of hospital stay, placenta praevia, uterine rupture, and neonatal respiratory morbidity (*NICE*, 2004; *Caesarean section*: CG13).

42. Answer A

Diabetes during pregnancy is associated with an increased risk of miscarriage, pre-eclampsia, preterm labour, fetal macrosomia, congenital malformations, birth injury, stillbirth, neonatal hypoglycaemia, induction of labour, or Caesarean section (*NICE*, 2008; *Diabetes in pregnancy*: CG63).

43. Answer B

According to NICE (2007; *Heavy menstrual bleeding*: CG44), heavy menstrual bleeding should be defined as excessive menstrual blood loss interfering with the woman's physical, emotional and social quality of life. A biopsy is indicated for persistent intermenstrual bleeding and in women ≥45 years where treatment has been ineffective. The levonorgestrel-releasing intrauterine system is a first-line treatment for menorrhagia (NICE, 2007). Norethisterone may be used from days 5 to 26 of the menstrual cycle; long-acting progestogens may also be considered. Ferritin levels, hormone levels and thyroid function tests are not recommended by NICE.

44. Answer D

Fluoxetine is the selective serotonin reuptake inhibitor with the lowest known risk during pregnancy. Citalopram and fluoxetine are found in breast milk at relatively high levels. Sertraline is found in breast milk at a relatively low level. Selective serotonin reuptake inhibitors may be associated with an increased risk of persistent neonatal pulmonary hypertension if taken after 20 weeks of gestation (*NICE*, 2007; *Antenatal and postnatal mental health*: CG45).

45. Answer A

All people ≥16 years are presumed to have capacity to consent, unless there is evidence to suggest otherwise. A competent person is able to understand and retain information relevant to their decision about their care; a competent person is able to weigh up risks and benefits relating to their decision. According to the Fraser guidelines, a doctor may give contraceptive advice or treatment if the following criteria are fulfilled: a girl (<16 years) has capacity to make decisions, that the patient cannot be persuaded to inform her parents, that she is likely to have sexual intercourse with or without contraceptive treatment, that unless she is given advice/treatment her physical or mental health would be at risk, and giving treatment is in her best interests.

46. Answer **B**

Levonorgestrel is effective if taken within 72 hours of unprotected sexual intercourse. It may be used between 72 and 120 hours but this is unlicensed. Levonorgestrol is less effective than the insertion of an intrauterine device; ulipristal is as effective as levonorgestrel. Following emergency hormonal contraception, barrier contraception needs to be used until the next period. A copper intrauterine contraceptive device can be inserted up to 120 hours after unprotected sexual intercourse.

47. Answer **C**

There is no limit on gestational age when considering termination of pregnancy if there is a risk to the mother's life or if the fetus is likely to be born with severe physical or mental abnormalities. If the continuance of the pregnancy would involve risk of injury to the physical or mental health of the pregnant woman or any existing child(ren), an abortion may be performed up to 24 weeks.

48. Answer **E**

Hypothyroidism occurs in approximately 2.5% of pregnant women. Hypothyroidism in pregnancy is treated with a larger dose of thyroxine when compared with the non-pregnant state. Postpartum thyroiditis presents 3–6 months postpartum and it is usually painless. Those with postpartum thyroiditis usually test positive for thyroid peroxidise antibodies, but treatment is not usually required. During pregnancy there is an increase in thyroid-binding globulin and albumin.

49. Answer **FFFTT**

According to the NHS Cervical Screening Programme, all women between the ages of 25 and 64 are eligible for cervical screening. Between the ages of 25 and 49 screening is every 3 years and up to the age of 64 screening is every 5 years in England. It is recommended that women over the age of 65 are screened if there has been a recent abnormal smear or screening has not taken place since the age of 50. If a woman has never been sexually active, the risk of cervical cancer is low. HPV 16 and 18 are associated with cervical cancer. Smoking increases the risk of cervical cancer.

50. Answer **FTFTT**

There is no evidence that pregnancy accelerates HIV progression. The major obstetric factors that may increase perinatal transmission of HIV include: vaginal delivery in the absence of HAART, duration of membrane rupture, chorioamnionitis and preterm delivery (*RCOG*, 2010; *Green-top Guideline 39: Management of HIV in pregnancy*). Routine universal antenatal screening for HIV is a part of antenatal care in developed countries. Sexual health screening is advisable in a high-risk patient. Increased HIV replication in the genital tract secondary to local infection may increase the risk of vertical transmission. Pregnant women who are HIV-positive may reduce the risk of mother-to-child transmission from about 35% to 2% by using HAART, avoiding breastfeeding and elective Caesarean section.

51. Answer **TTTTT**

Galactorrhoea usually refers to milky secretion from the breast that is not related to breastfeeding. Nipple stimulation or suckling will produce physiological galactorrhoea. Possible causes include prolactinomas, acromegaly, Cushing's disease, chronic renal failure, liver failure and conditions that may cause pituitary stalk or hypothalamic infiltration. Medications such as antihypertensives, phenothiazine antipsychotics, antidepressants (particularly selective serotonin re-uptake inhibitors), or combined oral and depot contraceptives may be the underlying cause. Illicit drugs such as cannabis and opiates may also be responsible.

52. Answer **TTTTT**

An ectopic pregnancy is one that occurs at any site apart from the endometrium. The majority of ectopic pregnancies occur in the Fallopian tubes. In a significant proportion of women risk factors such as previous ectopic pregnancy, a history of infertility, endometriosis, previous Fallopian tube surgery and/or salpingitis are present. Haemoperitoneum may cause referred shoulder tip pain. If serial measurements of β-hCG levels are falling, expectant management may be an option as some ectopic pregnancies may resolve spontaneously. Salpingectomy and salpingostomy may be performed both by laparoscopy or laparotomy. If the Fallopian tube is irreparably damaged or diseased, salpingectomy is the preferred procedure as there is a significant risk of recurrence of ectopic pregnancy in that tube.

53. Answer **TFTTF**

Fibroids or leiomyomata are benign myometrial tumours that occur in up to 30% of women. Furthermore, these tumours are found in up to 80% of uteri at autopsy. Fibroids are more common in African and Afro-Caribbean women, non-smokers and in women who delay pregnancy voluntarily or involuntarily. Most women with fibroids are asymptomatic. Fibroids may be associated with menorrhagia, pelvic pain, pressure symptoms and subfertility. Furthermore, pregnant women have an increased risk of fibroid degeneration, abnormal fetal lie and postpartum haemorrhage.

54. Answer **TTFTT**

PID describes infection and inflammation of the upper genital tract; this may involve the endometrium, Fallopian tubes and/or ovaries, as well as the surrounding peritoneum. On occasion this may lead to Fitz–Hugh–Curtis syndrome where infection spreads along the upper peritoneum to the liver capsule causing perihepatic 'violin string' adhesions. Generally PID is caused by a cervical sexually transmitted infection, usually as a result of ascending infection with *Chlamydia trachomatis* and *Neisseria gonorrhoeae.* Bimanual examination is likely to reveal adnexal tenderness and cervical excitation. With a single episode of PID, the incidence of subfertility is 20% due to tubal and ovarian adhesions.

55. Answer **TFFFF**

Highly effective contraception in women with epilepsy is particularly important due to the risk of congenital malformation with anti-epileptic drugs (AEDs). Furthermore, seizure control and AED pharmacokinetics may change during pregnancy. Although folate levels may not decline with all AEDs, those with epilepsy are advised to supplement their intake. Contraceptive failure is a risk in women taking oral contraceptives with AEDs that induce microsomal enzymes in the liver, such as cytochrome P450. Enzyme-inducing AEDs include carbamazepine, ethosuximide, phenytoin and topiramate. In women taking liver enzyme-inducing drugs who are considering using the combined oral contraceptive pill, a regimen using at least 50 mcg of oestrogen is recommended. Additional contraceptive cover such as a barrier method is recommended for 4 weeks after a liver enzyme-inducing medication is stopped.

56. Answer **FTTTF**

Hyperemesis gravidarum refers to a severe intractable nausea and vomiting that usually occurs between 8 and 12 weeks of pregnancy in up to 2% of patients. Hyperemesis may result in dehydration with electrolyte imbalance and alkalosis. There may be nutritional deficiencies and weight loss. Women with hyperemesis are more likely to have a baby that is small for gestational age and has a low birth weight. Hyperemesis gravidarum may be associated with this condition in a previous pregnancy, multiple gestations, trisomy 21 and prior or current molar pregnancy. Although thyroid function tests are commonly carried out, hyperthyroidism causing nausea and vomiting is rare.

57. Answer **FFTFF**

In neonatal resuscitation, the airway is opened with the baby on his/her back with the head in the neutral position. The ratio of compressions to inflations is 3:1. Stimulation may be provided by drying the baby. Five inflation breaths are given if breathing is inadequate at 90 seconds. Aspirating meconium from the baby's nose and mouth while the head is on the perineum is no longer recommended (Resuscitation Council, 2005).

58. Answer FTTTT

Pre-eclampsia is a multisystem disorder causing widespread vascular endothelial dysfunction, occurring beyond the 20th week of gestation. It is associated with raised blood pressure and proteinuria in a previously normotensive woman. Central nervous system features include eclampsia or seizures and cerebral haemorrhage. Other features may include pulmonary oedema, renal tubular necrosis, jaundice and HELLP syndrome (haemolysis, elevated liver enzymes and lowered platelets).

59. Answer TFTTT

Risk factors for venous thromboembolism in pregnancy include thrombophilia, antithrombin deficiency, protein C and S deficiency, systemic lupus erythematosus, inflammatory bowel disease, nephrotic syndrome, age >35 years, BMI >30 kg/m², smoking, pre-eclampsia, prolonged labour and Caesarean section (*RCOG*, 2007; *Green-top Guideline 28: Thromboembolic disease in pregnancy and the puerperium*).

60. Answer FFTTT

Folic acid supplementation is recommended prior to conception until the 12th week of pregnancy to reduce the risk of neural tube defects. For most women the dose is 400 mcg daily but a higher dose is recommended if epilepsy medications are being taken. Vitamin D supplementation (10 mcg/day) is recommended for all pregnant women especially those at higher risk, for example, South Asians and those with limited exposure to sunlight. In women who are overweight, weight loss is advised to reduce the risk of pregnancy complications such as pre-eclampsia. Immunity to rubella (German measles) should be checked prior to pregnancy ideally.

61. Answer FFFFT

Varicella zoster virus (VZV) is a DNA virus of the herpes family that is transmitted by respiratory droplets and by direct personal contact. Chickenpox is infectious 48 hours before the rash appears and continues to be infectious until the vesicles crust over 5 days later. 90% of the antenatal population in the UK are seropositive for VZV immunoglobulin antibody. Antibodies may be checked in those with uncertain history of previous infection but national screening does not take place. If a pregnant woman not immune to VZV has been exposed, immunoglobulin may be given up to 10 days after contact (*RCOG*, 2007; *Green-top Guideline 13: Chickenpox in pregnancy*).

62. Answer **TFTTF**

Counselling for sterilisation should include a discussion of risks and benefits associated with other long-term reversible methods of contraception. Women who request tubal occlusion postpartum should be made aware of the increased regret rate and the possible increased failure rate. The lifetime risk of failure in tubal occlusion is approximately 1 in 200. The failure rate for vasectomy is 1 in 2000 after clearance has been given. Women should be advised to use contraception until the day of surgery and to continue to use it until their next menstrual period. A pregnancy test is performed before the operation to exclude the possibility of a pregnancy, a negative test does not exclude the possibility of a luteal-phase pregnancy. A man is considered sterile when he has produced two consecutive semen samples with no spermatozoa; this is usually 3 months post-vasectomy. (*RCOG*, 2004; *Evidence-based Clinical Guideline 4: Male and female sterilisation*).

63. Answer **FFTTF**

Antenatal screening includes testing for anaemia, red cell allo-antibodies, hepatitis B virus, HIV, syphilis and immunity against rubella (*NICE*, 2008; *Antenatal care: routine care for the healthy pregnant woman*: CG62).

64. Answer **TFFFF**

Combined oral contraceptives may be used to treat dysmenorrhoea and menorrhagia. Fibroids are less likely to be symptomatic and there are fewer functional ovarian cysts with the combined oral contraceptive pill. There is a reduced risk of ovarian and endometrial cancer. Emergency contraception is recommended if two or more combined oral contraceptive pills are missed from the first seven tablets in a packet and there has been unprotected sexual intercourse. Vomiting and diarrhoea can interfere with the absorption of the pill; if vomiting occurs within 2 hours of taking the combined oral contraceptive pill, another pill should be taken as soon as possible.

65. Answer **TTTFT**

Sacral nerve stimulation is recommended for the treatment of UI in women who have not responded to conservative treatments. Retropubic mid-urethral tape procedures are recommended for stress UI where conservative management has failed. Women with microscopic haematuria (if aged 50 years and older) or visible haematuria should be referred urgently (*NICE*, 2006; *Urinary incontinence*: CG40).

66. Answer **TTFFF**

Planned Caesarean section should be offered to women with: term singleton breech (if external cephalic version has failed or is contraindicated), twin pregnancy where the first twin is breech, HIV, primary genital herpes in the 3rd trimester, and grade 3 and 4 placenta praevia (*NICE*, 2004; *Caesarean section*. CG13).

67. Answer **TFFFF**

Ideally folic acid supplements are recommended from pre-conception until 12 weeks of gestation. It is advised to stop oral hypoglycaemic agents except metformin and commence insulin if required. Alternative antihypertensives to angiotensin-converting enzyme inhibitors and angiotensin-II receptor antagonists should be considered. Statins are not recommended during pregnancy as congenital anomalies have been reported (*BNF*).

68. Answer **TFFFT**

Risk factors for postpartum haemorrhage include: placenta praevia, multiple pregnancy, pre-eclampsia, obesity, delivery by emergency Caesarean section, operative vaginal delivery, prolonged labour >12 hours, age >40 years (*RCOG*, 2009; *Green-top Guideline 52: Prevention and management of postpartum haemorrhage*).

69. Answer **FFTFF**

Approximately 60% of term and 80% of preterm babies develop jaundice in the first week of life. Up to 10% of breastfed babies may still be jaundiced at 4 weeks. Jaundice is prolonged if it occurs for more than 14 days in term babies and for more than 21 days in preterm babies. Physiological jaundice occurs when the baby is 2–3 days old as a result of increased red blood cell breakdown and immature liver function (*NICE*, 2010; *Neonatal jaundice*: CG98).

70. Answer **FFTTF**

Large amounts of epidural opioid may cause short-term respiratory problems in the newborn. It is associated with a longer second stage of labour and an increased risk of instrumental vaginal delivery. It is not associated with a longer first stage of labour or an increased risk of Caesarean section (*NICE*, 2007; *Intrapartum care*: CG55).

71. Answer **TTFFF**

Obesity in pregnancy is associated with an increased risk of thromboembolism, gestational diabetes, pre-eclampsia, postpartum haemorrhage, Caesarean section and fetal congenital anomaly (*CMACE/RCOG*, 2010; Joint Guideline: *Management of women with obesity in pregnancy*).

72. Answer **FFFTF**

Neisseria gonorrhoeae is a Gram-negative diplococcus that is transmitted by inoculation of infected secretions between mucous membranes. The incubation period is usually up to 7 days. Most men present with a urethral discharge or dysuria; rectal and pharyngeal infection may present in men who have sex with other men. Women are often asymptomatic but may present with vaginal discharge or symptoms of PID.

73. Answer **FTTFT**

The underlying genetic basis for Down syndrome is trisomy 21 in most cases; it may also arise as a result of translocations and mosaicism. Maternal age is a risk factor, for example the risk may be approximately 1:400 at 35 years and 1:30 at 45 years. Features of Down syndrome include hypotonia, oblique palpebral fissures, brachycephaly, epicanthic folds and single palmar creases. Down syndrome is associated with duodenal atresia, congenital heart disease, cataracts, hypothyroidism, acute myeloblastic and lymphoblastic leukaemia.

74. Answer **TFTTF**

Anaemia in pregnancy may be the result of haemodilution due to the increase in plasma volume; it is commonly iron deficiency anaemia. Women are screened for anaemia at the booking visit and at 28 weeks. Anaemia is confirmed by Hb <11 g/dl at the booking visit. Oral iron therapy may cause nausea and altered bowel habit. Iron preparations are better absorbed on an empty stomach but may be taken with food to reduce the risk of side effects.

75. Answer **TTFFF**

Intrauterine growth restriction (IUGR) may be related to hypertension, fetal alcohol syndrome, maternal smoking, thrombophilia, pre-eclampsia, toxoplasmosis and rubella infections. Asymmetric growth restriction where abdominal girth is reduced and where head circumference is relatively preserved may occur where there is placental insufficiency. There is usually symmetric growth restriction in the case of chromosomal abnormality. Oligohydramnios may be suggestive of IUGR.

76. Answer **TFFTT**

Parvovirus B19 is a droplet infection that may also be transmitted through blood products. The incubation period is 13–18 days. The presence of a 'slapped cheek' rash indicates lack of infectivity. It may cause an aplastic crisis. Infection during 4–20 weeks of gestation may cause fetal hydrops.

77. Answer **TFFFT**

Group B streptococcus may cause severe early onset of infection in the neonate; risk factors include prolonged rupture of membranes, prematurity and intrapartum pyrexia (*RCOG*, 2003; *Green-top Guideline 36: Prevention of early onset neonatal group B streptococcal disease*). Routine antenatal screening is not carried out in the UK. Penicillin G is recommended for intrapartum prophylaxis, and clindamycin is recommended in those who are penicillin-allergic.

78. Answer **TFFTT**

During the menopause there is a reduction of ovarian follicular activity and this causes a decline in oestrogen and progesterone levels. There is a subsequent increase in luteinising and follicle stimulating hormone. Symptoms include menstrual irregularity, hot flushes, vaginal dryness, loss of libido and mood changes. Measuring hormone levels may be helpful in the diagnosis of premature menopause.

79. Answer **FFTFT**

Hydatidiform moles may be complete or partial. Partial moles consist of two sets of paternal haploid genes and one set of maternal haploid genes, whereas complete moles are diploid and consist of paternal genetic material. Complete moles do not contain fetal tissue. Multiple pregnancy, previous molar pregnancy and pregnancy at the extremes of reproductive age are risk factors for molar pregnancy. Ultrasonography demonstrating a 'snow storm' appearance is usually diagnostic. Clinical features include vaginal bleeding, hyperemesis, early pre-eclampsia and large-for-dates. Molar pregnancies are registered because follow-up is required.

80. Answer **FFFTF**

Blood is returned from the placenta by the umbilical vein to the inferior vena cava; the ductus venosus acts as a conduit for most of this blood. The foramen ovale shunts oxygenated blood from the right to the left atrium. Blood is diverted from the pulmonary trunk into the descending aorta through the ductus arteriosus. Closure of the foramen ovale is brought about by pressure changes in the atria. This arises at birth when the lungs expand and there is increased blood flow in the pulmonary arteries. There is functional closure of the ductus arteriosus caused by contraction of the muscular wall. Fetal haemoglobin has an oxygen dissociation curve that is shifted to the left when compared with adult haemoglobin.

81. Answer **FTFFT**

Sickle cell disease is a chronic haemolytic disorder that is autosomal recessive. Sickle cell disease in pregnancy increases the risk of intrauterine death, low birth weight and IUGR. Screening should ideally be preconceptual or by at least 8–10 weeks of pregnancy. In the neonate symptoms of sickle cell anaemia may present when levels of fetal haemoglobin decline. Features include anaemia, jaundice and an increased risk of infection with encapsulated bacteria.

82. Answer **FFFFT**

The following are risk factors for developmental dysplasia of the hip (DDH): family history, female sex, breech presentation, oligohydramnios and prematurity. Screening for this condition forms part of the neonatal and 6 week examination. Ultrasound is not used routinely as a screening tool in the UK. The Barlow test attempts to displace the hip by applying backward pressure to the head of the femur. The Ortolani test applies forward pressure to the femoral heads to relocate a dislocation or subluxation.

83. Answer **FFTFT**

According to the World Health Organization, prematurity is defined as being born before 37 weeks gestation. Risk factors for prematurity include: pre-eclampsia, multiple pregnancy, polyhydramnios, and smoking. Premature babies have an increased risk of hypothermia, hypoglycaemia, respiratory distress syndrome, neonatal jaundice and intraventricular brain haemorrhage. Premature babies may receive immunisations according to their chronological age.

84. Answer **TFTFF**

HIV may cause a seroconversion illness 1–6 weeks after infection. Screening for other sexually transmitted infections is important. The window period refers to the time when markers of HIV infection are undetectable. Universal testing for HIV is recommended in sexual health clinics and in drug dependency programmes. There is universal antenatal testing of HIV in the UK. Testing usually involves an assay for HIV antibody and p24 antigen. The British HIV Association (2008) advises that the window period may only be 1 month for fourth generation assays. Point of care tests from a fingerprick or mouth swab sample have a low specificity and the British HIV Association recommends that all positive results from point of care tests are confirmed by serology.

85. Answer **FFFTF**

HRT is associated with an increased risk of endometrial, breast and ovarian cancer. The risk of breast cancer is increased within 1–2 years of being on HRT. The additional risk of breast cancer associated with HRT declines within 5 years of stopping HRT. In women aged 50–59 years there are six additional cases of breast cancer per 1000 women using combined HRT for 5 years. There are 24 additional cases of breast cancer per 1000 women aged 50–59 years using combined HRT for 10 years.

86. Answer **TTFFF**

Vasectomy is less invasive when compared with female sterilisation which requires intra-abdominal access. The lifetime risk of failure in tubal occlusion in women is approximately 1 in 200. The failure rate for vasectomy is 1 in 2000 after clearance has been given. A man is considered sterile post-vasectomy when he has produced two consecutive semen samples with no spermatozoa; this is usually 3 months post-vasectomy (*RCOG*, 2004; *Evidence-based Clinical Guideline 4: Male and female sterilisation*.). Vasectomy does not increase the risk of testicular cancer.

87. Answer **TTFTF**

Women may be advised that if they are less than 6 months postpartum, amenorrhoeic and fully breastfeeding, the lactational amenorrhoea method is over

98% effective in providing contraception. Breastfeeding delays ovulation. The risk of pregnancy is increased when night feeds are stopped, menstruation starts and there is not exclusive breastfeeding. Breastfeeding is associated with mother-to-child transmission of HIV.

88. Answer **FTTFF**

NuvaRing (combined vaginal ring) is licensed for contraceptive use. It is a latex-free, flexible ring that is 54 mm in diameter. The ring is inserted into the vagina by the patient for 3 weeks per cycle, after this there is a ring-free week (analogous to the combined oral contraceptive pill-free interval). It may remain *in situ* during tampon use and sexual intercourse. The rings are stored in a refrigerator prior to dispensing to a patient. After dispensing, it is advised that the rings are stored at room temperature for no longer than 4 months.

Exam paper 2

Extended matching questions

Options for questions 1–3

A	Hyperemesis gravidarum	**F**	Irritable bowel syndrome
B	Gastroenteritis	**G**	Appendicitis
C	Ovarian cyst accident	**H**	Early onset pre-eclampsia
D	Fibroid degeneration	**I**	Pulmonary embolus
E	Urinary tract infection	**J**	Ovarian hyperstimulation syndrome

Instructions: for each of the patients described below, choose the **single** most appropriate diagnosis from the list above. Each option may be used once, more than once or not at all.

Question 1	A 32 year old woman had an embryo transfer 1 week ago; she self-referred to the A&E department with shortness of breath, abdominal discomfort and vomiting.
Question 2	A 43 year old woman self-referred to the A&E department with sudden onset of right lower abdominal pain, nausea and an episode of vomiting. She has an appendicectomy scar and was very tender in the right fornix on pelvic examination.
Question 3	A 26 year old woman self-referred to the A&E department feeling generally unwell and vomiting. She had a normal early pregnancy scan at 8 weeks. Her liver enzymes were raised.

Options for questions 4–6

A	Oxytocin for augmentation	F	Fetal blood sampling
B	Await spontaneous labour within 24 hours	G	Dexamethasone
C	Await normal delivery	H	Erythromycin
D	Instrumental delivery	I	Emergency Caesarean section
E	Elective Caesarean section	J	Re-examine after 1 hour

Instructions: for each of the case histories described below, choose the **single** most appropriate action from the list above. Each option may be used once, more than once or not at all.

Question 4	A 30 year old primigravida attended labour ward at 38 weeks. She had premature rupture of membranes 6 hours ago.
Question 5	A multigravida in her 6th pregnancy has a delayed second stage labour of 2 hours. She has been pushing for more than 1 hour with adequate uterine contractions. The cardiotocograph is reassuring, the head is high.
Question 6	A 26 year old primigravida attended the delivery suite in spontaneous labour at 38 weeks. Her labour has progressed well. She received an epidural and has been fully dilated for 2 hours. She has been pushing for more than 1 hour and now feels exhausted. The head is visible and the cardiotocograph is reassuring.

Options for questions 7–9

A	Gonadotrophin-releasing hormone analogues	F	Mirena IUS (LNG-IUS)
B	Mifepristone	G	Depo-Provera
C	Danazol	H	Gestrinone
D	Tranexamic acid	I	Misoprostol
E	Combined oral contraceptive pill	J	Cyclical progesterone orally

Instructions: for each of the cases described below, choose the **single** most appropriate contraceptive from the list above. Each option may be used once, more than once or not at all.

Question 7	A 31 year old P2+0 plans to go travelling for a few weeks; she admits that she is forgetful with pills. Her last pregnancy was with a 'coil' *in situ*. Her recent pelvic scan was reported to be normal.
Question 8	A 26 year old with a long-standing history of dysmenorrhoea and menorrhagia had a laparoscopy and was diagnosed with endometriosis. She is keen to conceive in a few months.
Question 9	A 45 year old woman had an endometrial biopsy for irregular bleeding. This showed endometrial hyperplasia without atypia.

Options for questions 10–12

A	Atonic postpartum haemorrhage	F	Uterine rupture
B	Cervical trauma	G	Cervical shock
C	Retained products of conception	H	Aspirin
D	Bleeding disorder	I	Disseminated intravascular coagulation
E	Infection	J	Therapeutic anticoagulation

Instructions: for each of the cases described below, choose the **single** most appropriate option from the list above. Each option may be used once, more than once or not at all.

Question 10	A 36 year old multigravida had severe abdominal pain and collapsed after delivery. She has had two previous Caesarean sections.
Question 11	A 32 year old multigravida had an uneventful pregnancy and labour, after delivery she developed heavy vaginal bleeding.
Question 12	A 29 year old primigravida had a twin delivery where delivery of the placenta was difficult. She was discharged home and re-admitted 1 week later with heavy vaginal bleeding.

Options for questions 13–15

A	Nuchal translucency scan and human chorionic gonadotrophin	F	Human chorionic gonadotrophin and unconjugated oestriol
B	Nuchal translucency scan, human chorionic gonadotrophin, pregnancy-associated plasma protein A, alpha-fetoprotein, unconjugated oestriol and inhibin A	G	Nuchal translucency scan, human chorionic gonadotrophin, alpha-fetoprotein, unconjugated oestriol and inhibin A
C	Human chorionic gonadotrophin and alpha-fetoprotein	H	Nuchal translucency scan, human chorionic gonadotrophin and pregnancy-associated plasma protein A
D	Nuchal translucency scan	I	Human chorionic gonadotrophin, alpha-fetoprotein and unconjugated oestriol
E	Unconjugated oestriol and inhibin A	J	Human chorionic gonadotrophin, alpha-fetoprotein, unconjugated oestriol and inhibin A

Instructions: for each of the Down syndrome tests described below, choose the **single** most appropriate range of investigations from the list above. Each option may be used once, more than once or not at all.

Question 13	Components of the integrated test for antenatal screening of Down syndrome
Question 14	Components of the combined test for first trimester screening of Down syndrome
Question 15	Components of quadruple test for second trimester screening of Down syndrome

Options for questions 16–18

A	Androgen insensitivity syndrome	F	Turner syndrome
B	Polycystic ovarian syndrome	G	Asherman syndrome
C	Premature ovarian failure	H	Resistant ovary syndrome
D	Mayer–Rokitansky–Kuster–Hauser syndrome	I	Anorexia nervosa
E	Kallmann syndrome	J	Hyperprolactinaemia

Instructions: for each of the patients described below, choose the **single** most appropriate diagnosis from the list above. Each option may be used once, more than once or not at all.

Question 16	An 18 year old with normal secondary sexual characteristics seeks advice for primary amenorrhoea. She has cyclical pelvic pain. Her BMI is 23. Her sisters had menarche at 12 years.
Question 17	A 15 year old presented with primary amenorrhoea. She is 1.65 metres tall and has Tanner IV breast development. She has no pubic or axillary hair.
Question 18	A 25 year old presented with secondary amenorrhoea. She is the shortest of her siblings and has a webbed neck. Her sense of smell is normal.

Options for questions 19–21

A	Squamous metaplasia	**F**	Moderate dyskaryosis
B	Cervical erosion	**G**	Borderline nuclear changes
C	Cervical polyp	**H**	Arias–Stella change
D	Mild dyskaryosis	**I**	Severe dyskaryosis
E	Cervical wart	**J**	Nabothian cysts

Instructions: for each of the patients described below, choose the **single** most appropriate diagnosis from the list above. Each option may be used once, more than once or not at all.

Question 19	A 45 year old woman was referred by her GP with an unusually 'bumpy' cervix. There is no intermenstrual or post-coital bleeding. A cervical smear 6 months ago was normal. Examination demonstrated multiple pearly white spots on the ectocervix.
Question 20	A 28 year old was referred with recurrent post-coital bleeding and copious clear vaginal discharge. Examination revealed a circumferential red area around the cervical os with contact bleeding.
Question 21	A 25 year old was referred to the colposcopy clinic with previous inadequate smears. There was an irregular sessile growth on the cervix. Similar growths were visualised on the vaginal wall

Options for questions 22–24

A	Repeat fetal blood sampling within 10 minutes	F	Caesarean section
B	Wait and watch	G	Repeat fetal blood sampling within 30 minutes
C	Fetal blood sampling	H	Stop oxytocin
D	Urgent delivery	I	Subcutaneous terbutaline
E	Instrumental delivery	J	Real-time ultrasonography

Instructions: for each of the situations described below, choose the **single** most appropriate action from the list above. Each option may be used once, more than once or not at all.

Question 22	A 30 year old woman during labour undergoes cardiotocography. The trace shows a fetal heart rate of 106 beats/minute and variability of less than 5 beats/minute for 50 minutes.
Question 23	A 32 year primigravida is admitted in labour. Cardiotocography shows a fetal heart rate of 190 beats/minute. Fetal blood sampling shows pH values of 7.21–7.24.The trace remains the same after 15 minutes.
Question 24	Fetal blood sampling done for a pathological trace shows pH ≤7.2.

Options for questions 25–27

A	Shelf pessary	F	Abdominal hysterectomy
B	Reassurance	G	Abdominal hysterectomy and colposuspension
C	Pelvic floor exercises	H	Anterior and posterior repair
D	Vaginal hysterectomy	I	Combined procedure
E	Pelvic floor repair	J	Sacrospinous fixation

Instructions: for each of the patients described below, choose the **single** most appropriate treatment from the list above. Each option may be used once, more than once or not at all.

Question 25	An 88 year old lady has a history of a lump inside the vagina which is getting worse. She has a history of chronic asthma and unstable angina. On examination there is a second degree uterovaginal prolapse and a large cystocele.
Question 26	A 30 year lady presents with urinary incontinence on coughing and laughing since the birth of her child 6 months ago.
Question 27	A 45 year old lady presents with a 3 year history of a lump inside her vagina. The lump is causing discomfort and she is unable to use tampons. She also has a long-standing history of troublesome menorrhagia. She is unable to cope with the symptoms and would like a permanent solution.

Options for questions 28–30

A	Depo-Provera and condom use	F	Nexplanon
B	Progestogen-only pill	G	Continue the combined oral contraceptive pill
C	Continue using barrier contraception	H	Stop the combined oral contraceptive pill
D	NuvaRing	I	Stop using barrier contraception
E	HRT	J	Depo-Provera only

Instructions: for each of the patients described below, choose the **single** most appropriate contraceptive option from the list above. Each option may be used once, more than once or not at all.

Question 28	A 40 year old woman has recently been diagnosed with breast cancer; she has been taking the combined oral contraceptive pill for the last 3 years.
Question 29	A 26 year old HIV-positive woman on nevirapine therapy would like to choose the most suitable method of contraception.
Question 30	A 47 year old woman with amenorrhoea for 1 year has been using barrier contraception.

Single best answer questions

31 Which one of the following statements about physiological changes in pregnancy is **true**?

A   Thyroxine-binding globulin levels decrease during pregnancy.

B   Venous return in the inferior vena cava is helped by lying in the right lateral position.

C   Tidal volume increases during pregnancy.

D   Gastrointestinal motility is increased.

E   Creatinine clearance is reduced.

32 Which one of the following statements about Rhesus status is **false**?

A   Rhesus D-negative women who give birth to a Rhesus-positive baby should be offered anti-D 72 hours after delivery.

B   Sensitisation to the Rhesus antigen does not occur with external cephalic version.

C   Sensitisation to the Rhesus antigen may occur after chorionic villus biopsy.

D   For routine antenatal prophylaxis NICE recommends that two doses of anti-D immunoglobulin should be given at 28 and 34 weeks of gestation.

E   For routine antenatal prophylaxis NICE recommends that a single dose of anti-D immunoglobulin may be given between 28 and 30 weeks of gestation.

33 Which one of the following statements about genital mutilation is **false**?

A   Female genital mutilation is a child protection issue.

B   Keloid scar formation may result from female genital mutilation.

C   Urinary outflow obstruction may result from female genital mutilation.

D It is an offence for any person to excise or mutilate any part of the labia majora or clitoris of another person in England, Scotland and Wales.

E Female genital mutilation is prohibited by law in England, Scotland and Wales, if committed against a UK national.

34 Concerning thromboprophylaxis in pregnancy, which one of the following statements is **false**?

A Low molecular weight heparins may be used for antenatal thromboprophylaxis.

B Low molecular weight heparins should be stopped during labour.

C Low molecular weight heparins are safe during breastfeeding.

D Low molecular weight heparins for 7 days after delivery should be considered for mothers with BMI >40 kg/m^2.

E Women with antiphospholipid syndrome should be offered thromboprophylaxis antenatally and for 7 days after delivery.

35 Which one of the following statements is **true**?

A The Rotterdam diagnostic criteria for polycystic ovary syndrome do not include clinical signs of hyperandrogenism.

B Hyperprolactinaemia does not cause oligomenorrhoea.

C Total testosterone level may be normal in women with PCOS.

D Luteinising hormone (LH)/follicle-stimulating hormone (FSH) ratios are helpful in diagnosing PCOS.

E Polycystic ovaries have to be present to make the diagnosis.

36 Which one of the following statements regarding postpartum haemorrhage is **true**?

A Primary postpartum haemorrhage is the loss of ≥500 ml of blood from the genital tract up to 48 hours postnatally.

B Secondary postpartum haemorrhage is abnormal or excessive bleeding from the genital tract up to 7 days postnatally.

C The risk of postpartum haemorrhage may be reduced by active management in the third stage of labour.

D Secondary postpartum haemorrhage is not associated with endometritis.

E Obesity is not a risk factor for postpartum haemorrhage.

37 Which one of the following statements regarding premenstrual syndrome (PMS) is **true**?

A PMS regularly occurs during the follicular phase of the menstrual cycle.

B Cognitive behavioural therapy is not helpful in severe PMS.

C Continuous low dose selective serotonin re-uptake inhibitors are not helpful in PMS.

D Luteal phase low dose selective serotonin re-uptake inhibitors are not helpful in PMS.

E The combined oral contraceptive pill may be helpful for severe PMS.

38 Regarding postnatal care, which one of the following statements is **false**?

A In seronegative women who have been given the MMR (measles, mumps and rubella) vaccine postnatally, pregnancy should be avoided for 1 month.

B In seronegative women who have been given the MMR vaccine postnatally, breastfeeding should be avoided.

C Newborn hearing screening takes place within 4–5 weeks.

D The newborn examination is performed within 72 hours.

E The newborn blood spot test is usually carried out when the baby is 5–8 days old.

39 Regarding breastfeeding, which one of the following statements is **false**?

A The Department of Health recommends exclusive breastfeeding for the first 4 months of an infant's life.

B Breastfeeding increases the risk of mother-to-child transmission of human immunodeficiency virus.

C Breastfeeding may continue whilst receiving appropriate antibiotics for mastitis.

D Breast infections are commonly caused by *Staphylococcus aureus.*

E Tongue-tie may make breastfeeding difficult.

40 Concerning genital herpes in pregnancy, which one of the following statements is **true**?

A For women presenting with a primary episode of genital herpes at the time of delivery, Caesarean section is not recommended.

B For women presenting with a primary episode of genital herpes within 6 weeks of their due date, Caesarean section is recommended.

C For women presenting with a recurrent episode of genital herpes at the time of delivery, Caesarean section is recommended.

D Neonatal herpes is not caused by herpes simplex virus type 1.

E Neonatal herpes is not caused by herpes simplex virus type 2.

41 Concerning recurrent miscarriage, which one of the following statements is **true**?

A Recurrent miscarriage refers to the loss of two or more pregnancies.

B Peripheral blood karyotyping may be helpful in investigating recurrent miscarriage.

C Women diagnosed with recurrent miscarriage do not need a pelvic ultrasound scan.

D Women diagnosed with recurrent miscarriage should routinely have thyroid function tests.

E Screening for bacterial vaginosis with 2nd trimester miscarriage is not essential.

42 Regarding placenta praevia, which one of the following statements is **true**?

A Transvaginal ultrasound should not be used to diagnose placenta praevia.

B Women with major placenta praevia who have previously bled should be managed as inpatients from 32 weeks of gestation.

C Placenta praevia typically presents with the sudden onset of painful bleeding.

D Previous Caesarean section is not associated with placenta praevia.

E Advanced maternal age is associated with placenta praevia.

43 Which one of the following statements about physiological changes in pregnancy is **true**?

A Glomerular filtration rate decreases.

B Alkaline phosphatase deceases.

C Leukocytosis occurs during pregnancy.

D Serum iron increases.

E Bilirubin increases.

44 Which one of the following statements regarding fertility is **false**?

A Infertility refers to the failure to conceive after regular unprotected intercourse for 1 year in the absence of known reproductive pathology.

B Semen analysis and an assessment of ovulation should be made prior to making an assessment of tubal occlusion.

C Lifestyle advice for couples wishing to conceive may include advice concerning folic acid.

D Lifestyle advice for couples wishing to conceive includes advising intercourse every 2–3 days.

E Lifestyle advice for couples wishing to conceive includes smoking cessation.

45 Which one of the following statements regarding chlamydia is true?

A   Chlamydia is caused by a Gram-positive bacteria.

B   Chlamydia is always symptomatic.

C   Chlamydia never presents with a reactive arthritis.

D   Chlamydia is commonly diagnosed from a urethral swab in a man.

E   If a vaginal examination is indicated, an endocervical swab for chlamydia may be taken.

46 Which one of the following statements is true?

A   Follow-up retinal assessment for women with pre-existing diabetes should be performed at 24 weeks if there is diabetic retinopathy.

B   Retinal assessment for women with pre-existing diabetes should be performed after the first contact in pregnancy if it has not taken place in the last year.

C   Diabetes in pregnancy may be managed in a routine antenatal clinic.

D   Hypoglycaemia awareness is increased during pregnancy.

E   Diabetic retinopathy is stable during pregnancy.

47 Regarding the NHS Newborn Blood Spot Screening programme, which one of the following conditions is **not** screened for?

A   Phenylketonuria.

B   Tay–Sachs disease.

C   Medium-chain acyl-CoA dehydrogenase deficiency.

D   Cystic fibroisis.

E   Sickle cell disease.

48 Which one of the following statements regarding *Trichomonas vaginalis* is **true**?

A *Trichomonas vaginalis* is a bacterium.

B It is usually treated with azithromycin.

C Contact tracing is not required if *Trichomonas* infection is confirmed.

D *Trichomonas vaginalis* infection does not present with a frothy discharge.

E *Trichomonas* infection in men may cause a urethral discharge and dysuria.

Multiple choice questions

For each of these multiple choice questions, you must indicate which of the statements are true and which are false.

49 Concerning Bartholin's cysts and abscesses

   A Bartholin's glands are situated at the 2 o'clock and 10 o'clock position of the vestibule on either side of the vagina.

   B Bartholin's glands are usually palpable.

   C Bartholin's cysts or abscesses occur in approximately 10% of women.

   D Abscesses present as painless unilateral labial swellings.

   E Symptomatic cysts and abscesses may be managed by insertion of a balloon catheter.

50 Concerning congenital adrenal hyperplasia (CAH)

   A CAH is an autosomal dominant condition with variable penetrance.

   B It is commonly caused by 11-hydroxylase deficiency.

   C CAH forms part of the national neonatal screening programme.

   D Male babies may be identifiable as they usually have ambiguous genitalia.

   E Female babies usually present in adrenal crisis.

51 With regard to genitourinary prolapse

   A Increased parity is not a risk factor for genitourinary prolapse.

   B Obesity is a risk factor for genitourinary prolapse.

   C Prolapse does not present with urinary symptoms.

   D Prolapse may cause dyspareunia.

   E Constipation may occur as a result of genitourinary prolapse.

52 Concerning anaemia in pregnancy

A If haemoglobin is <10.5 g/dl antenatally, haemoglobinopathy does not need to be excluded.

B Parenteral iron should be used first-line for iron-deficiency anaemia.

C Pregnant women should have their blood group and antibody status checked at the booking visit.

D Pregnant women should have their blood group and antibody status checked at 18–20 weeks of gestation.

E Blood loss may be minimised during labour by active management of the second stage.

53 Regarding risks associated with diagnostic hysteroscopy

A The risk of serious complications arising from diagnostic hysteroscopy is approximately 2 women in every 100.

B There is a risk of uterine perforation with diagnostic hysteroscopy.

C Bladder damage frequently occurs with diagnostic hysteroscopy.

D Failure to instrument the uterus frequently occurs.

E Infection and bleeding rarely occur.

54 Regarding postmenopausal cysts and bleeding

A Ovarian cysts should be evaluated by transvaginal ultrasonography and CA19.9 levels.

B Simple unilateral cysts that are <6 cm diameter are considered to be at low risk of malignancy.

C Women presenting with postmenopausal bleeding not on hormone replacement therapy should be referred routinely to a specialist.

D Women taking tamoxifen who present with postmenopausal bleeding should be referred urgently to a specialist.

E Women with persistent or unexplained postmenopausal bleeding after stopping hormone replacement therapy for 8 weeks should be referred routinely to a specialist.

55 With regard to delaying menstruation

A If a woman is taking the combined oral contraceptive pill, menstruation is not delayed by omitting the pill-free interval.

B Norethisterone is usually taken once daily when used to delay menstruation.

C Norethisterone is usually taken approximately one week before the onset of menstruation is expected.

D Menstruation usually occurs 2–3 days after stopping norethisterone.

E Norethisterone may cause breast tenderness.

56 Concerning ovarian torsion

A Induction of ovulation as part of infertility treatment decreases the risk of ovarian torsion.

B Pregnancy may be associated with ovarian torsion.

C Ovarian torsion typically presents with a gradual onset of pain.

D Ectopic pregnancy may present with clinical features of ovarian torsion.

E Ovarian tumours decrease the risk of ovarian torsion.

57 Regarding HIV and pregnancy

A Pregnant women who are HIV positive should be offered sexual health screening.

B Vaginal delivery is absolutely contraindicated.

C If a woman chooses to undergo a vaginal delivery, artificial rupture of membranes should be avoided.

D The MMR vaccine is recommended in pregnant women who are HIV positive.

E Invasive diagnostic testing is always contraindicated in pregnant women who are HIV positive.

58 Concerning chickenpox and pregnancy:

A Chickenpox during pregnancy is a common cause of miscarriage.

B Chickenpox during pregnancy may cause severe maternal illness.

C Varicella vaccine can safely be given during pregnancy.

D If a pregnant woman not immune to Varicella zoster virus has been exposed, immunoglobulin may be given up to 7 days after contact.

E Pregnancy should be avoided for 3 months in a woman of reproductive age who has received the Varicella vaccine.

59 In management of ectopic pregnancy:

A Laparoscopic salpingectomy is preferred over laparoscopic salpingostomy if the Fallopian tube is damaged.

B Methotrexate is used in medical management.

C Medical management is offered to women with minimal symptoms and serum hCG <3000 IU/l.

D Ectopic pregnancy may be managed on an outpatient basis.

E Women with suspected ectopic pregnancy who are Rhesus negative do not need to be given anti-D immunoglobulin.

60 Concerning congenital diaphragmatic hernia

A A congenital diaphragmatic hernia is often the result of an anterior defect.

B Left-sided hernias allow herniation of the large and small bowel in the thoracic cavity.

C A congenital diaphragmatic hernia does not cause pulmonary hypoplasia.

D A congenital diaphragmatic hernia does not cause pulmonary hypertension.

E There is surfactant dysfunction in this condition.

61 Regarding antibiotics and pregnancy

A Metronidazole may be used in pregnancy.

B Ciprofloxacin may be safely used in pregnancy.

C Trimethoprim may be safely used in pregnancy.

D Amoxicillin may be used in pregnancy.

E Azithromycin may be used in pregnancy.

62 Concerning the 'Saving Mothers' Lives' report

A The Centre for Maternal and Child Enquiries produces biennial reports on enquiries into maternal deaths.

B The most recent report was for 2005–2008.

C The commonest cause of direct death was thromboembolism in the most recent report.

D The leading cause of indirect death was diabetes in the most recent report.

E The enquiry revealed that obesity was a risk factor for maternal mortality.

63 With regard to toxic shock syndrome (TSS)

A TSS may cause a diffuse or erythrodermic rash.

B TSS commonly presents with hypertension.

C TSS does not cause gastrointestinal symptoms.

D Uterine packing after postpartum haemorrhage is not a risk factor for TSS.

E Postpartum sepsis is a risk factor for TSS.

64 Concerning multiple pregnancy

A Advanced maternal age is not associated with multiple pregnancy.

B A family history of dizygotic twins is associated with multiple pregnancy.

C Race is not associated with multiple pregnancies.

D There is a risk of multiple pregnancy with ovulation induction.

E Multiple pregnancy is not associated with an increased risk of prematurity.

65 Regarding peripartum cardiomyopathy

A Peripartum cardiomyopathy generally occurs up to 1 year postpartum.

B Peripartum cardiomyopathy is usually associated with pre-existing heart disease.

C Multiparity is not a risk factor for peripartum cardiomyopathy.

D This condition is a hypertrophic cardiomyopathy.

E Ankle oedema may be associated with peripartum cardiomyopathy as well as the later stages of pregnancy.

66 Concerning criteria for screening programmes

A Screening may take place for an important clinical condition with an early asymptomatic stage where there is a benefit in early detection.

B The screening test carried out should be validated and acceptable to those being screened.

C The screening test carried out should be validated and acceptable to health care professionals.

D There should be evidence that early treatment is as beneficial as late treatment of the condition.

E A screening programme always results in a reduction in morbidity and mortality.

67 The following are absolute contraindications for the combined oral contraceptive pill:

A BMI above 30 kg/m^2 AND history of superficial thrombophlebitis.

B Smoking AND aged over 30 years.

C   Venous thromboembolism in a sister aged 30 AND smoking.

D   Blood pressure above systolic 160 mmHg or diastolic 95 mmHg.

E   Diabetes AND smoker.

68   Regarding statistics

A   The absolute risk reduction is not the same as the difference between the risk of an event in the control group and the risk of the event in the intervention group.

B   The number needed to harm refers to how many people need to have an intervention for one person to benefit from it.

C   The number needed to treat may be calculated if the absolute risk reduction is known.

D   A positive predictive value is obtained by calculating the proportion of people who have a positive test result who actually have the disease.

E   If the relative risk is 1 there is a difference between an intervention and control group.

69   Regarding definitions

A   If a woman dies during pregnancy or up to 28 days postpartum from an obstetric cause or a cause exacerbated by pregnancy, this may be classified as a maternal death.

B   A direct maternal death may occur postpartum.

C   An indirect cause of maternal death may have been exacerbated by pregnancy.

D   A neonatal death is where a live-born baby dies before 42 completed days.

E   The perinatal mortality rate refers to the number of stillbirths and neonatal deaths per 1000 live births.

70 Concerning androgen insensitivity syndrome

A Androgen insensitivity syndrome is an autosomal recessive condition.

B There is phenotypic male development in a chromosomally female patient.

C Patients with androgen insensitivity syndrome have normal testes.

D Patients with androgen insensitivity syndrome have a womb.

E This condition may present with secondary amenorrhoea.

71 Krukenberg tumours:

A Are primary ovarian tumours.

B Have the breast as the commonest primary site.

C Are mostly unilateral.

D Mostly occur through transcoelomic spread.

E Often display signet ring cells on histology.

72 Regarding cervical screening

A Cervical screening may be postponed by 3 months following pregnancy.

B Cervical screening is best performed mid-cycle.

C Women who have never been sexually active do not need cervical screening.

D Women in a same-sex relationship do not need cervical screening.

E Women must attend their GP surgery for cervical screening to ensure continuity of care.

73 Concerning HIV and pregnancy

A Elective Caesarean section may reduce the risk of vertical transmission.

B Artificial rupture of membranes should be avoided.

C Breastfeeding should be recommended in the UK.

D   Polymerase chain reaction is used for the diagnosis of infant infections.

E   Zidovudine prophylaxis in the neonate may reduce vertical transmission.

74   Regarding management of fibroids

A   Tranexamic acid may relieve symptoms.

B   Gonadotrophin releasing hormone (GnRH) analogues increase the size of fibroids.

C   Fibroids may be managed hysteroscopically.

D   Fibroids may be treated by occlusion of the uterine arteries.

E   There is a 50% risk of fibroid recurrence.

75   Concerning cytomegalovirus (CMV) and pregnancy

A   CMV is a herpes virus.

B   CMV is not found in saliva.

C   CMV infection in pregnancy does not cause intrauterine growth restriction.

D   CMV infection in pregnancy may cause conductive hearing loss.

E   CMV infection in pregnancy may cause hepatosplenomegaly.

76   Regarding epilepsy and contraception

A   Levetiracetam does not affect the efficacy of the combined oral contraceptive pill.

B   Lamotrigine does not affect the efficacy of the combined oral contraceptive pill.

C   The progestogen-only pill in epilepsy has reduced efficacy with enzyme-inducing AEDs.

D   Depot medroxyprogesterone acetate (DMPA) is unaffected by liver enzyme-inducing drugs.

E   The Mirena coil is a potential contraceptive option for women on enzyme-inducing medications.

77 Risk factors for pre-eclampsia include:

A Previous pre-eclampsia.

B Primagravida.

C Family history of pre-eclampsia.

D Hydatidiform mole.

E BMI <35 kg/m^2.

78 Concerning Caesarean section

A Bladder or ureteric injury commonly occurs during Caesarean section.

B Emergency hysterectomy is a rarely occurring risk during Caesarean section.

C There is a decreased risk of uterine rupture in subsequent pregnancies following Caesarean section.

D There is a decreased risk of placenta praevia in subsequent pregnancies following Caesarean section.

E There is an increased risk of Caesarean section when vaginal delivery is attempted following a previous Caesarean section.

79 Regarding alcohol and pregnancy

A Alcohol misuse during pregnancy is associated with low birth weight.

B Fetal alcohol syndrome is associated with facial anomalies.

C Newborns with fetal alcohol syndrome commonly display withdrawal.

D Pre-conceptual screening for substance misuse may be considered.

E The diagnosis of fetal alcohol syndrome is often delayed.

80 Regarding pregnancy and lithium therapy

A There is an increased risk of fetal heart defects.

B Low levels of lithium are found in breast milk.

C Lithium therapy is safe during pregnancy.

D Women taking lithium therapy may have a home delivery if there is adequate support.

E Fluid status should be closely monitored during labour.

81 Hormone replacement therapy (HRT):

A Should be stopped in a patient that presents with sudden onset of shortness of breath.

B Should be stopped if there is unexplained unilateral lower leg swelling.

C Should be stopped if diastolic blood pressure is persistently >90 mmHg.

D Should be stopped if systolic blood pressure is persistently >140 mmHg.

E Does not need to be stopped if severe abdominal pain occurs.

82 Regarding risks associated with multiple pregnancy

A Multiple pregnancies are not associated with an increased risk of congenital abnormalities when compared with singleton pregnancies.

B There is an increased risk of oligohydramnios with multiple pregnancy.

C Hyperemesis gravidarum occurs more frequently in multiple pregnancy when compared with singleton pregnancy.

D There is a decreased risk of placental abruption with multiple pregnancy.

E There is a decreased risk of cord prolapse with multiple pregnancy.

83 Concerning medications which cause galactorrhoea

A Metoclopramide may cause galactorrhoea.

B Risperidone does not cause galactorrhoea.

C Tricyclic antidepressants do not cause galactorrhoea.

D Selective serotonin reuptake inhibitors may cause galactorrhoea.

E Cimetidine may cause galactorrhoea.

84 Regarding placental abruption

A There is an increased risk of placental abruption with advanced maternal age.

B Hypertension does not increase the risk of placental abruption.

C Prolonged rupture of membranes is not associated with an increased risk of placental abruption.

D Cocaine use may increase the risk of placental abruption.

E Cigarette smoking reduces the risk of placental abruption.

85 Concerning vaccination during pregnancy

A Haemophilis influenza type B (Hib) vaccine may be given during pregnancy.

B Yellow fever vaccine may be given during pregnancy.

C The MMR vaccine may be given during pregnancy.

D The BCG vaccine may be given during pregnancy.

E Meningococcal vaccines may be given during pregnancy.

86 Regarding bacterial vaginosis (BV)

A The presence of a smelly white discharge does not support the diagnosis of BV.

B Clue cells on microscopy support the diagnosis of BV.

C pH of vaginal fluid >5.5 is part of the Amsel criteria.

D The release of a fishy odour on addition of 10% potassium hydroxide may be used to diagnose BV.

E Intravaginal metronidazole gel may be used to treat BV.

87 Concerning treatment of UTIs during pregnancy

A UTIs may be treated with cephalosporins during pregnancy.

B Nitrofurantoin may be used to treat UTIs throughout pregnancy.

C Nitrofurantoin may be used to treat UTIs if a mother is breastfeeding.

D The teratogenic risk with trimethoprim is greatest in the second trimester.

E Ciprofloxacin may be safely used during pregnancy.

88 Regarding 5-alpha-reductase deficiency

A 5-alpha-reductase deficiency is an X-linked condition.

B 5-alpha-reducatase deficiency results in chromosomally female patients having ambiguous genitalia.

C Patients with this condition have normal testes.

D Patients with this condition have a womb.

E It may be difficult to distinguish androgen insensitivity syndrome from 5-alpha-reductase deficiency clinically.

Answers and explanations for exam paper 2

1. Answer J Ovarian hyperstimulation syndrome

Ovarian hyperstimulation syndrome may be caused by inducing ovulation for assisted conception. Symptoms of mild hyperstimulation occur during treatment cycles; however, moderate and severe symptoms usually occur 6–8 days after treatment ends. Mild symptoms include abdominal bloating and nausea. In moderate ovarian hyperstimulation syndrome, nausea and vomiting are more prominent features; women may report weight gain and an increase in abdominal girth. With increasing severity an increase in abdominal girth caused by ascites may result in shortness of breath. Other features include dehydration and an increased risk of venous thromboembolism.

2. Answer C Ovarian cyst accident

In the setting of acute pelvic pain, ovarian torsion forms part of the differential diagnosis. Significant haemorrhage of an ovarian cyst often manifests itself with an abrupt onset of pelvic pain. There may be haemorrhage into a corpus luteal cyst or follicular cyst. Cyst rupture may be associated with haemoperitoneum and hypotension, with the latter usually dominating the clinical picture.

3. Answer A Hyperemesis gravidarum

Hyperemesis gravidarum refers to severe and intractable nausea and vomiting that usually occurs between 8 and 12 weeks of pregnancy in up to 2% of pregnancies. In some patients symptoms may lessen but persist up to the 20th week of pregnancy and, in some cases, symptoms may occur throughout pregnancy. It is the most common reason for hospitalisation during early pregnancy. Hyperthyroidism causing nausea and vomiting is rare. Transient hyperthyroidism is seen in about 60% of women with hyperemesis, this usually resolves by 18 weeks of gestation. This may be caused by raised levels of hCG or hypersensitivity of thyroid hormone receptors to hCG. Elevated transaminases may occur in up to 25% of patients with hyperemesis gravidarum. This often resolves once the nausea has settled. Significantly elevated liver enzymes, however, may be a sign of another underlying liver condition such as hepatitis or liver injury. Amylase may be elevated in approximately 10% of patients with hyperemesis gravidarum.

4. Answer B Await spontaneous labour within 24 hours

Up to 60% of women with prelabour rupture of membranes (PROM) at term will go into labour within 24 hours. After 24 hours, induction of labour may be considered.

5. Answer I Emergency Caesarean section

In nulliparous women, delay in the active second stage of labour is diagnosed if it has lasted 2 hours. In multiparous women, delay in the active second stage of labour is diagnosed if it has lasted 1 hour. In this scenario there is a delayed second stage and the head is high therefore the most appropriate intervention is an emergency Caesarean section. Cephalopelvic disproportion is the most likely cause.

6. Answer D Instrumental delivery

In nulliparous women, delay in the active second stage of labour is diagnosed if it has lasted 2 hours. In this scenario the mother is tiring and the head is visible, therefore an instrumental delivery is the most appropriate option.

7. Answer G Depo-Provera

Depo-Provera is the most suitable option as the patient has tried the Mirena coil in the past and experienced a contraceptive failure with it. Furthermore this method is long-acting, reversible and not reliant on the patient remembering to take her contraception. Women should be counselled on risks and benefits of suitable contraceptive options prior to making a decision. Irregular bleeding is common with Depo-Provera but most women do become amenorrhoeic. Weight gain may cause discontinuation and there may be a delay in return of fertility. It may cause a reduction in bone mineral density in the first 2–3 years of use therefore its use should be re-evaluated. Progesterone-only contraception may be suitable for women with contraindications to the combined oral contraceptive pill.

8. Answer E Combined oral contraceptive pill

The combined oral contraceptive pill may be used to reduce menorrhagia and dysmenorrhoea caused by endometriosis. Suppression of ovarian function to improve pain related to endometriosis may be achieved by using the combined oral contraceptive pill, danazol, gestrinone, medroxyprogesterone acetate, and gonadotrophin-releasing hormone analogues. These treatment options have a variable side effect profile; the combined oral contraceptive pill represents the best option for this scenario.

9. Answer F Mirena IUS (LNG–IUS)

The Mirena intrauterine system is licensed for use as a contraceptive, for treatment of menorrhagia, and for endometrial protection if used with oestrogen hormone replacement therapy. It is effective in menorrhagia within 3–6 months of insertion as endometrial proliferation is prevented; bleeding usually becomes significantly lighter or may stop. Fertility is restored after removal. Enzyme-inducing medications are unlikely to reduce the contraceptive effect of the Mirena intrauterine system.

10. Answer **F** Uterine rupture

There is an increased risk of uterine rupture with trauma and previous Caesarean section or uterine surgery. Uterine rupture often does not present with typical signs. It may present with sudden severe pain, heavy vaginal bleeding, fetal distress and hypovolaemic shock. Uterine inversion may present with appearance of a vaginal mass, postpartum haemorrhage and hypovolaemic shock.

11. Answer **A** Atonic postpartum haemorrhage

Primary postpartum haemorrhage (PPH) is the loss of ≥500 ml of blood from the genital tract up to 24 hours postnatally. The risk of PPH may be reduced by active management in the third stage of labour and therefore prophylactic oxytocics are given. Uterine atony is a common cause of PPH. Risk factors for PPH include: placenta praevia, multiple pregnancy, pre-eclampsia, obesity, delivery by emergency Caesarean section, operative vaginal delivery, prolonged labour >12 hours and age >40 years. (*RCOG*, 2009; *Green-top Guideline 52: Prevention and management of postpartum haemorrhage.*)

12. Answer **C** Retained products of conception

Secondary PPH is abnormal or excessive bleeding from the genital tract between 24 hours and 12 weeks postnatally. Secondary PPH is often associated with endometritis or retained products of conception.

13. Answer **B** Nuchal translucency scan, hCG, PAPP-A, alpha-fetoprotein, unconjugated oestriol and inhibin A

From 11–13^{+6} weeks and 15–20 weeks, the integrated test includes the nuchal translucency scan, hCG, PAPP-A, alpha-fetoprotein, unconjugated oestriol and inhibin A.

14. Answer **H** Nuchal translucency scan, hCG and PAPP-A

From 11–13^{+6} weeks gestation the combined test may be performed. The combined test consists of the nuchal translucency scan, hCG and PAPP-A.

15. Answer **J** hCG, alpha-fetoprotein, unconjugated oestriol and inhibin A

The quadruple test may be carried out from 15–20 weeks. This includes hCG, alpha-fetoprotein, unconjugated oestriol and inhibin A.

16. Answer **D** Mayer–Rokitansky–Kuster–Hauser syndrome

Congenital absence of the vagina is a feature of Mayer–Rokitansky–Kuster–Hauser syndrome. This usually presents as primary amenorrhoea with normal secondary sexual characteristics because ovarian function is normal. As a result there may be cyclical abdominal pain without menstruation. Vaginal aplasia may be partial or complete. This condition may occur with other paramesonephric duct abnormalities; renal anomalies are often found.

17. Answer **A** Androgen insensitivity syndrome

Androgen insensitivity syndrome is a rare X-linked condition which may be partial or complete. Masculinisation of the external genitalia does not occur due to the loss of function mutation in the androgen receptor gene in a chromosomally male patient, therefore there is phenotypic female development. Patients with androgen insensitivity syndrome have normal testes. The testes produce anti-Mullerian hormone and this prevents development of the Fallopian tubes, uterus and upper vagina. This condition may present with primary amenorrhoea. Adolescents with androgen insensitivity syndrome may present with inguinal masses, that is, undescended testes. Furthermore, breast development is normal but they do not have pubic or axillary hair.

18. Answer **F** Turner syndrome

Turner syndrome is the most common sex chromosome abnormality in females. It may be caused by the absence of one X chromosome (45,X) or may result from mosaicism (for example, 45,X/46XX). Features include short stature, lymphoedema of the hands and feet at birth, gonadal dysgenesis, high palate, widely spaced nipples, wide carrying angle and a webbed neck. Cardiovascular features include an increased risk of coarctation of the aorta and a bicuspid aortic valve. It may present with primary or secondary amenorrhoea. Kallman syndrome is associated with a reduced or absent sense of smell with hypothalamic gonadotrophin-releasing hormone deficiency.

19. Answer **J** Nabothian cysts

Nabothian cysts are often asymptomatic and are seen as multiple translucent or yellow lesions on the cervix. They usually represent areas of tissue re-growth where the stratified squamous epithelium of the ectocervix has grown over columnar epithelium. This may cause obstruction to the cervical crypts.

20. Answer **B** Cervical erosion

An ectropion is caused when columnar epithelium extends around the external os. Cervical ectopy may be associated with puberty, pregnancy and oral contraceptive pill use. It is usually an asymptomatic condition but may present with bleeding and discharge.

21. Answer **E** Cervical wart

Genital warts are caused by different types of the human papilloma virus (HPV); they usually arise from direct skin contact during sexual intercourse. HPV types 6 and 11 are associated with genital warts. They may arise several months after infection. Barrier contraception may reduce the risk of HPV transmission. Genital warts may be multiple and may cause itching, bleeding or pain.

22. Answer **C** Fetal blood sampling

The baseline number of beats per minute and the variability of less than 5 beats per minute for 40–90 minutes in this scenario is non-reassuring. Fetal blood sampling should be considered.

23. Answer **G** Repeat fetal blood sampling within 30 minutes

pH ≥7.25 is normal, pH 7.21–7.24 is borderline and pH ≤7.20 is abnormal. In this scenario there is a borderline fetal blood sampling result. Sampling should be repeated within 30 minutes as the trace is pathological.

24. Answer **D** Urgent delivery

A fetal scalp blood pH level ≤7.20 is abnormal; therefore urgent instrumental or operative delivery is needed.

25. Answer **A** Shelf pessary

There is an increased risk of genitourinary prolapse with advancing age, vaginal delivery, increased parity and obesity. Prolapse may present with a sensation of pressure or fullness in the vagina, urinary symptoms, dyspareunia, constipation as well as incontinence. In this scenario an operative intervention is less desirable. Pessary insertion to reduce symptoms provides a suitable alternative provided that the perineum is able to hold a pessary in place. There is a risk of vaginal erosion, bleeding and infection that may be associated with pessary use.

26. Answer **C** Pelvic floor exercises

A trial of supervised pelvic floor muscle training of at least 3 months' duration should be offered to women with stress or mixed urinary incontinence. Pelvic floor exercises may stop deterioration where mild uterovaginal prolapse is present. However, it is unlikely that there will be an improvement with regards to any prolapse if this is already present.

27. Answer **D** Vaginal hysterectomy

In this scenario symptoms of uterovaginal prolaspe and menorrhagia may be improved by performing a vaginal hysterectomy. Vaginal hysterectomy is preferable to abdominal hysterectomy as this is associated with a shorter hospital stay and fewer complications.

28. Answer H Stop the combined oral contraceptive pill

The UK Medical Eligibility Criteria provide guidance for contraceptive use. Category 1 refers to a condition where there are no restrictions on contraceptive choice. In category 2 the advantages of a particular contraceptive option outweigh the disadvantages of using it. In category 3 the risks of a contraceptive option outweigh the benefits of using it. Category 4 refers to a condition where there is an unacceptable risk with an intervention. Use of the combined oral contraceptive pill is a category 4 intervention in the case of smoking ≥15 cigarettes/day, blood pressure ≥160/95, history of venous thromboembolism, protein C and S deficiencies, ischaemic heart disease, migraine with aura and current breast cancer.

29. Answer A Depo-Provera and condom use

The efficacy of the combined oral contraceptive pill, the progestogen-only pill and the progestogen-only implant may be reduced with antiretroviral drugs; therefore additional contraceptive cover is required. In women taking antiretroviral therapy, DMPA and intrauterine devices may be appropriate.

30. Answer C Continue using barrier contraception

In women >50 years, non-hormonal methods of contraception may be stopped after 1 year of amenorrhoea. In women <50 years, non-hormonal methods of contraception may be stopped after 2 years of amenorrhoea.

31. Answer C

Thyroxine-binding globulin levels increase during pregnancy. Venous return in the inferior vena cava may be compromised in late pregnancy in the supine position; pressure from the gravid uterus onto the inferior cava may be reduced by lying in the left lateral position. There is an increase in the minute ventilation during pregnancy due to an increase in tidal volume. Respiratory rate is unchanged during pregnancy. Gastrointestinal motility is decreased and constipation is common during pregnancy. Creatinine clearance is increased during pregnancy as a result of an increased glomerular filtration rate.

32. Answer B

All Rhesus D-negative women who give birth to a Rhesus-positive baby should be offered anti-D 72 hours after delivery. Sensitisation to the Rhesus antigen may occur after chorionic villus biopsy and external cephalic version. For routine antenatal prophylaxis NICE (2008; *Pregnancy (rhesus negative women) – routine anti-D*, TA156) recommends that two doses of anti-D immunoglobulin should be given at 28 and 34 weeks of gestation; alternatively a single dose may be given between 28 and 30 weeks of gestation (*BNF*).

33. Answer E

Female genital mutilation is a human rights and child protection issue. Late gynaecological complications of female genital mutilation include dyspareunia, chronic pain, recurrent UTIs, and urinary outflow obstruction. It is an offence for any person to excise or mutilate any part of the labia majora or clitoris of another person; no offence is committed if the surgery is related to labour or birth. Female genital mutilation committed against a permanent UK resident/UK national or abroad is prohibited by law in England, Scotland and Wales (*RCOG*, 2009; *Green-top Guideline 50: Female genital mutilation and its management*).

34. Answer E

Low molecular weight heparins may be used for antenatal thromboprophylaxis, but they should be stopped if there is vaginal bleeding and during labour. Low molecular weight heparins and warfarin are safe when breastfeeding. Low molecular weight heparins for 7 days after delivery should be considered for mothers with BMI >40 kg/m². Women with antiphospholipid syndrome should be offered thromboprophylaxis antenatally and for 6 weeks postpartum (*RCOG*, 2009; *Green-top Guideline 37: Reducing the risk of thrombosis and embolism during pregnancy and the puerperium*).

35. Answer C

According to the Rotterdam diagnostic criteria, polycystic ovary syndrome (PCOS) may be diagnosed if two out of three of the following criteria are present: oligomenorrhoea/amenorrhoea, clinical or biochemical signs of hyperandrogenism, polycystic ovaries on ultrasonography (defined as the presence of ≥12 follicles in at least one ovary). Other causes of oligomenorrhoea and amenorrhoea include premature ovarian failure, hypothyroidism and hyperprolactinaemia. Total testosterone level is normal to moderately elevated in women with PCOS. Luteinizing hormone (LH)/follicle-stimulating hormone (FSH) ratios are no longer considered useful in diagnosing PCOS (*RCOG*, 2007; *Green-top Guideline 33: Long-term consequences of polycystic ovary syndrome*).

36. Answer C

Primary postpartum haemorrhage (PPH) is the loss of ≥500 ml of blood from the genital tract up to 24 hours postnatally. Secondary PPH is abnormal or excessive bleeding from the genital tract between 24 hours and 12 weeks postnatally. The risk of PPH may be reduced by active management in the third stage of labour, therefore prophylactic oxytocics are given. Secondary PPH is often associated with endometritis (*RCOG*, 2009; *Green-top Guideline 52: Prevention and management of postpartum haemorrhage*). BMI >35 is a risk factor for PPH.

37. Answer E

Premenstrual syndrome (PMS) regularly occurs during the luteal phase of the menstrual cycle and symptoms disappear/significantly improve at the end of menstruation. Advice about stress reduction and exercise are helpful. The RCOG advise that continuous or luteal phase low dose selective serotonin re-uptake inhibitors as well as the combined oral contraceptive pill may be used as first line therapies in severe PMS (*RCOG, 2007; Green-top Guideline 48: Management of premenstrual syndrome*).

38. Answer B

In seronegative women who have been given the MMR (measles, mumps and rubella) vaccine postnatally, pregnancy should be avoided for 1 month (*NICE, 2006; Postnatal care, CG37*). In seronegative women who have been given the MMR vaccine postnatally, breastfeeding may continue. Newborn hearing screening takes place within 4–5 weeks, the newborn examination is performed within 72 hours, and the newborn blood spot test is usually carried out when the baby is 5–8 days old.

39. Answer A

The Department of Health recommends exclusive breastfeeding for the first 6 months of an infant's life. In the developed world, breastfeeding is not recommended in HIV-positive mothers. Breast infections are commonly caused by *Staphylococcus aureus;* breastfeeding may continue whilst receiving appropriate antibiotics for mastitis.

40. Answer B

Neonatal herpes is generally acquired as a result of contact with infected maternal secretions. For women presenting with a primary episode of genital herpes at the time of delivery or with n 6 weeks of their due date, Caesarean section is recommended. For those women who decline Caesarean section, rupture of membranes should be avoided. For women presenting with a recurrent episode of genital herpes at the time of delivery, Caesarean section is not recommended. Neonatal herpes may be caused by herpes simplex viruses type 1 and 2 as either virus may cause genital herpes (*RCOG, 2007; Green-top Guideline 30: Management of genital herpes in pregnancy*).

41. Answer B

Recurrent miscarriage refers to the loss of three or more pregnancies. Peripheral blood karyotyping is helpful in investigating recurrent miscarriage. Women diagnosed with recurrent miscarriage should have a pelvic ultrasound scan. The RCOG (2003; *Green-top Guideline 17: The investigation and treatment of couples with recurrent miscarriage*) advises that women diagnosed with recurrent miscarriage should not have routine thyroid function or glucose tests if they are asymptomatic. Screening for bacterial vaginosis with a history of preterm labour or 2nd trimester miscarriage may reduce the risk of further loss of pregnancy.

42. Answer **E**

If the placenta is partially or fully inserted into the lower segment of the uterus, placenta praevia is diagnosed. If the placenta overlies the cervical os, this represents a major praevia. Placenta praevia may be diagnosed on ultrasound scan, transvaginal ultrasound being more accurate than the transabdominal approach. Placenta praevia typically presents with the sudden onset of painless bleeding in the second or third trimester. Women with major placenta praevia who have previously bled should be managed as inpatients from 34 weeks of gestation. Advanced maternal age and previous Caesarean section are associated with an increased risk of placenta praevia (RCOG, 2005; *Green-top Guideline 27: Placenta praevia and placenta praevia accreta: diagnosis and management*).

43. Answer **C**

Serum iron decreases during pregnancy, transferrin and total iron binding capacity are increased. Alkaline phosphatase levels increase during pregnancy due to placental production whilst bilirubin levels decrease. Glomerular filtration rate is increased during pregnancy resulting in an increased creatinine clearance.

44. Answer **A**

Infertility refers to the failure to conceive after regular unprotected intercourse for 2 years in the absence of known reproductive pathology according to NICE (2004; *Fertility*, CG11). An assessment of ovulation may be made by taking a menstrual history and by measuring day 21 serum progesterone in a 28 day cycle as well as serum gonadotrophins. Lifestyle advice for couples wishing to conceive includes advising intercourse every 2–3 days, smoking cessation, keeping BMI <30, reducing alcohol intake and advising about recreational drug use (*NICE*, 2004; *Fertility*, CG11). Preconceptual care includes screening for rubella susceptibility, advising about folic acid use and cervical screening.

45. Answer **E**

Chlamydia is caused by an intracellular Gram-negative bacterium; it may be asymptomatic. Possible symptoms in women include vaginal discharge, lower abdominal pain, dyspareunia, intermenstrual or postcoital bleeding. Urethritis may be the presenting feature in men. Long-term complications include subfertility. It is an infection which may co-exist with other sexually transmitted infections. Chlamydial infection may result in urethritis, arthritis and conjunctivitis (Reiter's syndrome). A urethral swab in a male may be used to diagnose Chlamydia, however, this has been superseded by nucleic acid amplification tests on first void urine samples. In women, a self-administered vaginal swab may be taken; however, if an internal examination is performed usually an endocervical swab is taken.

46. Answer B

Diabetic retinopathy can worsen rapidly during pregnancy. Retinal assessment for women with pre-existing diabetes should be performed after the first contact in pregnancy if it has not taken place in the last year. Retinal assessment for women with pre-existing diabetes should then be performed at 16–20 weeks if there is diabetic retinopathy. If there is no diabetic retinopathy, the next assessment should be at 28 weeks. Women with insulin-treated diabetes should be advised that there is increased lack of awareness of hypoglycaemia in pregnancy especially in the first trimester. Diabetes in pregnancy should be managed in a joint diabetes and antenatal clinic (*NICE*, 2008; *Diabetes in pregnancy*, CG63).

47. Answer B

The NHS Newborn Blood Spot Screening programme includes testing for sickle cell disease, medium-chair acyl-CoA dehydrogenase deficiency, cystic fibrosis, phenylketonuria and congenital hypothyroidism. The blood spots are taken by heel prick. If a baby is thought to have one of these conditions, further tests are required.

48. Answer E

Trichomonas vaginalis is a protozoan. It may present with vulval itching, dysuria, abdominal pain and an offensive smelling yellow frothy discharge in women. Dysuria and discharge may be the presenting features in men. It is usually treated with metronidazole. As it is a sexually transmitted infection, contact tracing is important.

49. Answer FFFFT

Bartholin's glands are situated at the 4 o'clock and 8 o'clock position of the vestibule on either side of the vagina. The glands are not normally palpable. Bartholin's cysts or abscesses occur in approximately 2% of women. They usually occur in women who are nulliparous or of low parity. Cysts usually present with a painless labial swelling. Abscesses present acutely with a painful unilateral labial swelling. Symptomatic cysts and abscesses may be treated by incision and drainage, marsupialisation or by insertion of a balloon catheter.

50. Answer FFFFF

Congenital adrenal hyperplasia (CAH) is an autosomal recessive condition that is caused by an enzyme deficiency in the pathway for cortisol or aldosterone synthesis. It is commonly caused by 21-hydroxylase deficiency which results in cortisol deficiency; there may also be aldosterone deficiency and androgen excess with this. Neonatal screening is possible, but it is not carried out as part of the national screening programme. Female babies may be identifiable as they may have ambiguous genitalia with an enlarged clitoris in classic CAH. Females with salt-losing CAH are usually identified before a potential adrenal crisis. Males with salt-losing CAH may have no signs at birth and may therefore present with vomiting, failure to thrive or shock. Hyponatraemia, hyperkalaemia and/or hypoglycaemia may occur in adrenal insufficiency. Males that have a non-salt-losing form of this condition may present with virilisation at 2–4 years. Mild CAH in females may present later in childhood.

51. Answer **FTFTT**

There is an increased risk of genitourinary prolapse with advancing age, vaginal delivery, increased parity and obesity. Prolapse may present with a pressure sensation or fullness in the vagina, urinary symptoms, dyspareunia, constipation as well as incontinence.

52. Answer **FFTFF**

If haemoglobin is <10.5 g/dl antenatally and there is no evidence of haemoglobinopathy, haematinic deficiency should be considered. Oral iron should be used first-line for iron-deficiency anaemia. Parenteral iron may be considered if oral iron is not tolerated. Pregnant women should have their blood group and antibody status checked at booking and at 28 weeks. Blood loss may be minimised during labour by active management of the third stage.

53. Answer **FTFFF**

The risk of serious complications arising from diagnostic hysteroscopy is approximately 2 women in every 1000, according to the RCOG (2008; *Diagnostic hysteroscopy under general anaesthesia* (Consent Advice 1)). The risks associated with diagnostic hysteroscopy include uterine perforation, bladder or bowel damage and failure to instrument the uterus. Infection and bleeding are risks that occur more frequently.

54. Answer **FFFTF**

Ovarian cysts occur commonly in postmenopausal women. The RCOG recommend that ovarian cysts should be evaluated by transvaginal ultrasonography and CA125 levels (*RCOG*, 2003; *Green-top Guideline 34: Ovarian cysts in postmenopausal women*). Simple unilateral cysts that are <5 cm diameter are considered to be at low risk of malignancy. Women presenting with postmenopausal bleeding and not taking hormone replacement therapy, and those on tamoxifen with postmenopausal bleeding, should be referred urgently under the 2 week wait rule for further investigation. Women with persistent or unexplained postmenopausal bleeding after stopping hormone replacement therapy for 6 weeks should be referred urgently under the 2 week wait rule for further investigation (*NICE*, 2005; *Referral for suspected cancer*, CG27).

55. Answer **FFFTT**

If a woman is taking the combined oral contraceptive pill, menstruation may be delayed by taking the next pack directly and omitting the pill-free interval. Alternatively norethisterone may be used to delay menstruation. This is usually taken 3 times/day approximately 3 days before the onset of menstruation is expected. Menstruation usually occurs 2–3 days after stopping norethisterone. Side effects of norethisterone include bloating and breast tenderness.

56. Answer **FTFTF**

Ovarian torsion usually occurs in an enlarged ovary. Women undergoing induction of ovulation as part of infertility treatment are at increased risk of ovarian torsion. Ovarian tumours, previous history of pelvic surgery and pregnancy may be associated with ovarian torsion. Delayed diagnosis results in infarction and subsequent necrosis. Torsion typically presents with sudden, severe, unilateral abdominal pain which may be associated with nausea and vomiting. The differential diagnosis includes ectopic pregnancy, pelvic inflammatory disease and appendicitis.

57. Answer **TFTFF**

Routine universal antenatal screening for HIV is a part of antenatal care in developed countries. Sexual health screening is advisable in a high risk patient. According to the RCOG (2010; *Green-top Guideline 39: Management of HIV in pregnancy*), women with a detectable plasma viral load and/or who are not taking HAART should be offered elective Caesarean section to reduce the likelihood of vertical transmission. If a woman chooses to undergo a vaginal delivery after being appropriately counselled, artificial rupture of membranes and invasive procedures such as application of fetal scalp electrodes should be avoided. It is recommended that live vaccines such as MMR are avoided during pregnancy as there is a theoretical risk of fetal infection.

58. Answer **FTFFT**

90% of the antenatal population in the UK are seropositive for varicella zoster virus (VZV) immunoglobulin antibody. If a pregnant woman not immune to VZV has been exposed, immunoglobulin may be given up to 10 days after contact (*RCOG, 2007; Green-top Guideline 13: Chickenpox in pregnancy*). Varicella vaccine contains live attenuated virus and should be avoided during pregnancy. Pregnancy should be avoided for 3 months in a woman of reproductive age who has received the varicella vaccine. If chickenpox occurs in the first trimester, the risk of spontaneous miscarriage is not increased. However, if varicella infection occurs in the first 28 weeks of pregnancy there is a risk of fetal varicella syndrome.

59. Answer **TTTTF**

Management of ectopic pregnancy may involve salpingectomy or salpingostomy which may be performed both by laparoscopy or laparotomy. If the Fallopian tube is irreparably damaged or diseased, salpingectomy is the preferred procedure as there is a significant risk of recurrence of ectopic pregnancy in that tube. Methotrexate therapy may be appropriate for women with minimal symptoms and serum hCG <3000 IU/l. Women managed expectantly should have hCG measurements twice weekly and transvaginal ultrasound scans weekly; this may be done on an outpatient basis. Women with suspected ectopic pregnancy who are Rhesus negative should be given anti-D immunoglobulin.

60. Answer **FTFFT**

A congenital diaphragmatic hernia is caused by the diaphragm not fusing during fetal development; this often leads to a posterolateral defect. This condition results in pulmonary hypertension and hypoplasia as well as surfactant dysfunction. Most cases are diagnosed prenatally. Left-sided hernias allow herniation of the large and small bowel in the thoracic cavity. Right-sided hernias allow the liver and sometimes the large bowel to enter the thoracic cavity.

61. Answer **TFFTT**

Metronidazole may be used in pregnancy but the manufacturer advises avoiding high dose regimens. It is advised that quinolones are avoided during pregnancy as other antibiotics may be used more safely. Quinolones have been shown to cause arthropathy in animal studies. Trimethoprim should be avoided during pregnancy according to the manufacturer; there is a teratogenic risk in the first trimester. Azithromycin may be used in pregnancy but the manufacturer advises its use only if there are not suitable alternatives.

62. Answer **FFFFT**

The Centre for Maternal and Child Enquiries produces triennial reports on enquiries into maternal deaths. The most recent report was for 2006–2008 which was published in 2011. Maternal mortality refers to deaths of pregnant women as well as those 42 days postpartum. Direct deaths refer to those attributable to pregnancy or birth. The commonest cause of direct death was infection; many of these deaths were from community-acquired Group A streptococcal disease in 2006–2008. Indirect deaths are caused by pre-existing or new medical or mental health conditions exacerbated by pregnancy. The leading cause of indirect death was cardiac disease. The enquiry revealed that women who died had poorer health overall, were smokers and had a BMI >25.

63. Answer **TFFFT**

Toxic shock syndrome (TSS) occurs when toxin-secreting *Staphylococci* and *Streptococci* activate an inflammatory response. Risk factors include tampon use, gynaecological infections, postpartum sepsis and uterine packing after postpartum haemorrhage. TTS usually manifests with fever, a diffuse or erythrodermic rash, hypotension, vomiting and diarrhoea.

64. Answer **FTFTF**

Advanced maternal age, a family history of dizygotic twins and infertility treatment such as ovulation induction are associated with multiple pregnancy. Race may be associated with multiple pregnancy, for example, the incidence of multiple pregnancy is higher is Africa compared to the incidence in Asia.

65. Answer **FFFFT**

Peripartum cardiomyopathy refers to the development of cardiac failure in the last month of pregnancy up to 5 months postpartum. Most cases present within the first month postpartum. Before the last month of pregnancy there is generally no evidence of heart disease. Advancing maternal age and multiparity are risk factors. Shortness of breath on exertion and ankle oedema may be associated with peripartum cardiomyopathy as well as the later stages of pregnancy. Peripartum cardiomyopathy may cause chest pain, cough and paroxysmal nocturnal dyspnoea. This condition is a dilated cardiomyopathy that causes left ventricular dysfunction.

66. Answer **TTTFF**

Screening may take place for an important clinical condition with an early asymptomatic stage where there is a benefit in early detection. The test as well as the proposed treatment carried out should be validated and acceptable to those being screened. Both of these should be clinically and ethically acceptable to the public as well as healthcare professionals. There should be evidence that early detection and therefore early treatment is beneficial when compared with late management of the condition. Screening to allow identification of an important clinical condition should result in a reduction of morbidity and mortality.

67. Answer **TFTTT**

Smoking and age over 35 years would be an absolute contraindication to the combined oral contraceptive pill. If two of the following risk factors for arterial disease are present, the combined oral contraceptive pill should be avoided: family history of arterial disease in a first degree relative aged under 45 years, diabetes, hypertension, smoking, age >35 years, obesity and migraine (*BNF*). If two of the following risk factors for venous thromboembolism are present, the combined oral contraceptive pill should be avoided: family history of venous thromboembolism in a first degree relative aged under 45 years, known coagulation abnormality, obesity, immobility, history of superficial thrombophlebitis, age >35 years and smoking (*BNF*).

68. Answer **FFTTF**

The absolute risk reduction (ARR) refers to the difference between the risk of an event in the control group and the risk of the event in the intervention group. The number needed to treat (NNT) refers to how many people need to have an intervention for one person to benefit from it. The NNT may be calculated as the inverse of the absolute risk reduction. A positive predictive value is obtained by calculating the proportion of people who have a positive test result who actually have the disease. The relative risk evaluates how many times more likely it is that an event will occur in the intervention group when compared with the control group. If the relative risk is 1 there is no difference between the intervention and the control group.

69. Answer **FTTFF**

If a woman dies during pregnancy or up to 42 days postpartum from an obstetric cause or a cause exacerbated by pregnancy, this may be classified as a maternal death. A direct maternal death results from an obstetric complication of pregnancy, this may be postpartum. An indirect maternal death refers to a death attributable to a previous medical condition or a condition that developed during pregnancy that is not due to an obstetric cause. An indirect cause of maternal death may have been exacerbated by being pregnant. A neonatal death is where a live-born baby dies before 28 completed days. The number of neonatal deaths per 1000 live births is the neonatal death rate. The perinatal mortality rate refers to the number of stillbirths and neonatal deaths per 1000 live and stillbirths.

70. Answer **FFTFF**

Androgen insensitivity syndrome is a rare X-linked condition which may be partial or complete. Masculinisation of the external genitalia does not occur due to the loss of function mutation in the androgen receptor gene in a chromosomally male patient and therefore there is phenotypic female development. Patients with androgen insensitivity syndrome have normal testes. The testes produce anti-Mullerian hormone, this prevents development of the Fallopian tubes, uterus and upper vagina. This condition may present with primary amenorrhoea.

71. Answer **FFFFT**

Kruckenberg tumours are metastatic ovarian tumours that usually arise from stomach and colon malignancies. The stomach is the commonest primary site. Most tumours are bilateral and occur through lymphatic spread. Signet ring cells are typically found on histology.

72. Answer **TTFFF**

Cervical screening may be postponed by 3 months following pregnancy if there is a normal smear history. The cervical screening programme recommends that cervical screening is best performed mid-cycle. Women who have never been sexually active have a very low risk of cervical cancer. Women in a same-sex relationship are at low risk of cervical cancer; nevertheless, cervical screening is still recommended for both these groups. Women may attend their GP surgery or family planning / sexual health clinic for cervical screening.

73. Answer **TTFTT**

The risk of perinatal transmission of HIV can be minimised by preventing infant exposure to maternal blood and secretions. According to the RCOG (2010; *Green-top Guideline 39: Management of HIV in pregnancy*), women with a detectable plasma viral load and/or who are not taking HAART should be offered an elective Caesarean section to reduce the likelihood of vertical transmission. If a woman chooses to undergo a vaginal delivery after being appropriately counselled, artificial rupture of membranes and invasive procedures such as application of fetal scalp electrodes should be avoided. Episiotomy may increase the exposure of the infant to HIV during delivery and increase the risk of transmission (RCOG, 2010). Women should be advised to avoid breastfeeding even if taking antiretroviral therapy to avoid postnatal transmission. In the developing world this clearly depends on the availability and affordability of formula milk. Zidovudine prophylaxis is usually administered to the neonate.

74. Answer **TFTTF**

Tranexamic acid, which inhibits fibrinolysis, may be used for menorrhagia and mefenamic acid may be used to reduce inflammatory pain and uterine contractions. These treatments are useful when fibroids are relatively small and if periods are heavy and painful. Gonadotrophin-releasing hormone (GnRH) analogues are mainly used pre-operatively to reduce the size of the fibroids. If fibroids are mainly intracavity/submucosal, they may be resected hysteroscopically with good long-term results for fertility and menorrhagia. Uterine artery embolisation involves occluding the uterine arteries, usually with polyvinyl alcohol beads using a transfemoral approach (under local anaesthesia and light sedation), thereby impairing blood supply to the fibroids and causing shrinkage and necrosis over a few weeks. The risk of fibroid recurrence ranges from 15 to 30%.

75. Answer **TFFFT**

Cytomegalovirus (CMV) is the most common congenitally acquired infection; it is a DNA virus that is part of the herpes family. The virus may be found in breast milk, cervical secretions, saliva and blood products. CMV infection during pregnancy may cause intrauterine growth restriction. In 10% of fetuses with congenital infection it may also cause retinitis, hepatosplenomegaly, sensorineural hearing and visual loss. There is a risk for long term sequelae in those that are asymptomatic at birth.

76. Answer **TFTTT**

AEDs that do not affect the efficacy of the combined oral contraceptive pills include: gabapentin, levetiracetam, lamotrigine and valproate. However, it is known that lamotrigine clearance is increased in the presence of combined oral contraceptive pills and progestogen derivatives. This would reduce the efficacy of contraception and seizure control. The progestogen-only pill is not recommended by manufacturers as the efficacy is reduced with enzyme-inducing AEDs. However, DMPA is unaffected by liver enzyme-inducing drugs. The copper intrauterine device and the Mirena (levonorgestrel-releasing intrauterine system) coil are potential options for women on enzyme-inducing medications.

77. Answer **TTTTF**

Those women with a previous pregnancy complicated by severe pre-eclampsia have a high risk of recurrence in subsequent pregnancies for any type of pre-eclampsia. Risk factors include: age less than 20 years or more than 35 years, black race and BMI >35 kg/m^2.

78. Answer **FTFFT**

Bladder or ureteric injury and emergency hysterectomy are rarely occurring risks during Caesarean section. There is an increased risk of uterine rupture and placenta praevia in subsequent pregnancies following Caesarean section. There is an increased risk of Caesarean section when vaginal delivery is attempted following a previous Caesarean section.

79. Answer **TTFTT**

Fetal alcohol syndrome may be associated with characteristic facial anomalies, intrauterine growth restriction as well as cognitive impairment or learning disabilities. Alcohol withdrawal in neonates is uncommon but may present with agitation, tremors and seizures. The diagnosis of fetal alcohol syndrome may be delayed; it may present later with behavioural and cognitive problems.

80. Answer **TFFFT**

Lithium therapy during pregnancy is associated with an increased risk of cardiac defects. High levels of lithium are found in breast milk and lithium therapy should be avoided if possible during pregnancy, especially in the first trimester. However, lithium therapy may be continued despite the increased risk of cardiac defects if a woman is at high risk of relapse. Women taking lithium therapy should deliver in hospital because of the risk of dehydration and lithium toxicity (*NICE*, 2007; *Antenatal and postnatal mental health*, CG45).

81. Answer **TTFFF**

According to the *BNF*, HRT should be stopped if there is severe chest pain, suspicion of deep vein thrombosis or pulmonary embolus, severe abdominal pain, severe headache with neurological symptoms, jaundice, prolonged immobility post-operatively and blood pressure >160 systolic or >95 diastolic.

82. Answer **FFTFF**

Multiple pregnancies are associated with an increased risk of prematurity as well as an increased risk of congenital abnormalities when compared with singleton pregnancies. Multiple pregnancies are associated with an increased rate of maternal complications such as pre-eclampsia, anaemia, polyhydramnios and hyperemesis gravidarum. Furthermore, delivery may be complicated by an increased risk of malpresentation, operative delivery, placental abruption and cord prolapse.

83. Answer **TFFTT**

The following medications may cause galactorrhoea: metoclopramide, phenothiazines, risperidone, selective serotonin reuptake inhibitors, tricyclic antidepressants and cimetidine.

84. Answer **TFFTF**

There is an increased risk of placental abruption in women with a previous history of placental abruption, increased maternal age, hypertension, abdominal trauma, cigarette smoking, cocaine use and prolonged rupture of membranes. It is thought that cocaine use increases the risk of placental abruption by causing vasospasm.

85. Answer **TFFFT**

It is recommended that live vaccines are avoided during pregnancy as there is a theoretical risk of fetal infection (if there is significant exposure to a disease the benefits of vaccination may outweigh the risks). Inactivated vaccines may be given to pregnant women if protection is needed without delay. Haemophilis influenza type B (Hib) and meningococcal vaccines may be given during pregnancy. Yellow fever, BCG and MMR are live vaccines.

86. Answer **FTFTT**

Bacterial vaginosis (BV) may be diagnosed if at least 3 out of the 4 Amsel criteria are met. The Amsel criteria include: thin white discharge, clue cells on microscopy, pH of vaginal fluid >4.5 and release of a fishy odour on addition of 10% potassium hydroxide. Oral metronidazole, intravaginal metronidazole gel or clindamycin cream may be used to treat symptomatic women.

87. Answer **TFFFF**

Urinary tract infections (UTIs) may be treated with cephalosporins during pregnancy. Nitrofurantoin may be used to treat UTIs during pregnancy, but it is best avoided at term due to the risk of neonatal haemolysis. Breastfeeding should also be avoided in mothers taking nitrofurantoin because of the risk of neonatal haemolysis in glucose-6-phosphate dehydrogenase deficiency. Manufacturers of trimethoprim recommend avoiding it in pregnancy. There is a teratogenic risk with trimethoprim in the first trimester as it is a folate antagonist. Ciprofloxacin is best avoided during pregnancy as there are alternative regimens available for the treatment of UTIs.

88. Answer **FFTFT**

5-alpha-reductase deficiency is an autosomal recessive condition where testosterone is not converted to dihydrotestosterone. Dihydrotestosterone is needed for the masculinisation of the external genitalia in males. 5-alpha-reductase deficiency results in chromosomally male patients having ambiguous genitalia. Patients with this condition have normal testes that produce anti-Mullerian hormone and so the Fallopian tubes, uterus and the upper vagina do not develop. The epididymis, vas deferens and seminal vesicles are present. It may be difficult to distinguish androgen insensitivity syndrome from 5-alpha-reductase deficiency clinically. A child with 5-alpha-reductase deficiency may begin to virilise rather than feminise in puberty.

Exam paper 3

Extended matching questions

Options for questions 1–3

A	Blood transfusion	**F**	Serum ferritin
B	Folic acid and oral iron	**G**	B_{12} deficiency
C	Injectable iron and folic acid	**H**	Haemoglobin electrophoresis
D	Folic acid 400 mcg daily	**I**	Infection screen
E	Intravenous iron infusion	**J**	Iron deficiency anaemia

Instructions: for each of the case histories described below, choose the **single** most appropriate option from the list above. Each option may be used once, more than once or not at all.

Question 1	A multigravida is seen in antenatal clinic at 32 weeks; her haemoglobin is 8 g/dl. She feels very tired and is not taking her iron tablets regularly.
Question 2	A primigravida of African origin booked at 12 weeks of pregnancy. Her routine blood tests reveal that she is anaemic.
Question 3	A multigravida woman in her 4th pregnancy is found to be anaemic at 28 weeks of pregnancy. She feels breathless and tired.

Options for questions 4–6

A	Anti-D is not recommended	**F**	Anti-D is recommended
B	High dose anti-D	**G**	Anti-D immunoglobulin should be given at 28 weeks.
C	Anti-D immunoglobulin should be given at 34 weeks	**H**	Anti-D administration 72 hours after delivery
D	Fetal blood sampling	**I**	Immediate amniocentesis at a tertiary referral centre
E	Check middle cerebral artery peak systolic velocity	**J**	Delivery before 36 weeks

Instructions: for each of the case histories described below, choose the **single** most appropriate option from the list above. Each option may be used once, more than once or not at all.

Question 4	A 18 year old primigravida who is 6 weeks pregnant had minimal vaginal spotting, which has stopped. She is Rhesus negative.
Question 5	A 30 year old primigravida undergoes chorionic villus sampling. She is Rhesus negative.
Question 6	A 32 year old Rhesus-negative mother has anti-D antibodies detected at 24 weeks. She has rising antibody titres. The fetus is growing well.

Options for questions 7–9

A	Abdominal ultrasound	**F**	Intravenous antibiotics
B	Hormone replacement therapy	**G**	*In vitro* fertilisation
C	Mid-stream urine for culture and microscopy	**H**	Intrauterine insemination
D	Subcutaneous heparin	**I**	Nasogastric tube and intravenous fluids
E	Diagnostic laparoscopy	**J**	Hormonal profile (FSH, LH, oestradiol)

Instructions: for each of the patients described below, choose the **single** most appropriate management option from the list above. Each option may be used once, more than once or not at all.

Question 7	A 55 year old woman had an uncomplicated abdominal hysterectomy 2 days ago. Her temperature is 38°C. There is nil on systemic review and physical examination is unremarkable.
Question 8	A 27 year old nulliparous woman has had deep dyspareunia for 2 years. Her symptoms are getting worse and she has developed dysmenorrhoea recently. She is keen to conceive.
Question 9	A 50 year old woman had a total abdominal hysterectomy and left ovarian cystectomy 18 months ago. She has hot flushes and is tearful most of the time.

Options for questions 10–12

A	Risk greater than 1 in 150	F	Admit to hospital
B	Risk greater than 1 in 300	G	Transvaginal ultrasound
C	Antibiotics and stop breastfeeding	H	Antibiotics and continue breastfeeding
D	Abscess aspiration	I	Reassurance only
E	Topical oestrogen	J	No intervention

Instructions: for each of the patients described below, choose the **single** most appropriate option from the list above. Each option may be used once, more than once or not at all.

Question 10	A 24 year old primigravida had a spontaneous vaginal delivery 2 days ago and has developed a temperature. She has been breastfeeding and is now aware of left breast discomfort.
Question 11	A 28 year old woman underwent screening for Down syndrome at 11 weeks. She wants to know the threshold for diagnostic testing.
Question 12	A 60 year old woman had minimal vaginal bleeding for a day. There have been no further episodes of this.

Options for questions 13–15

A	Cervical carcinoma	F	CIN 3
B	Cervical polyp	G	Endometrial cancer
C	Atrophic endometrium	H	Choriocarcinoma
D	Ovarian cancer	I	Vulval cancer
E	Lichen sclerosus	J	Threatened miscarriage

Instructions: for each of the case histories described below, choose the **single** most appropriate diagnosis from the list above. Each option may be used once, more than once or not at all.

Question 13	A 60 year old woman has a 7 day history of vaginal bleeding. She had a left mastectomy 4 years ago and has been taking tamoxifen since then.
Question 14	A 66 year old woman had vaginal spotting and her transvaginal ultrasound scan showed that the endometrium was less than 4 mm. Tissue could not be obtained on endometrial aspiration. Her cervical smears have always been normal.
Question 15	A 40 year old multigravida has noticed intermenstrual and occasional postcoital bleeding. A recent smear test was normal. She is currently taking the combined oral contraceptive pill.

Options for questions 16–18

A	Expectant management	F	Reassurance
B	Medical management	G	Laparotomy
C	Laparoscopic salpingostomy	H	Urine pregnancy test
D	Laparoscopic salpingectomy	I	RU486
E	Potassium chloride	J	Misoprostol

Instructions: for each of the patients described below, choose the **single** most appropriate management option from the list above. Each option may be used once, more than once or not at all.

Question 16	A 30 year old woman is brought in by ambulance to the A&E department in a collapsed state. Her urine pregnancy test is positive.
Question 17	A 26 year old woman had a positive urine pregnancy test at 6 weeks. Her ultrasonography report is suggestive of a pregnancy of unknown location. Her β-hCG is 460 IU/l.
Question 18	A 25 year old woman is admitted with an ultrasound diagnosis of unruptured left tubal ectopic pregnancy. Cardiac activity is visualised.

Options for questions 19–21

A	Cervical dilatation	**F**	Anti-prostaglandins
B	Presacral neurectomy	**G**	Refer to psychiatrist
C	Laparoscopic sacral nerve ablation	**H**	Urine culture
D	Combined oral contraceptive pill	**I**	Irritable bowel syndrome
E	Hormone replacement therapy	**J**	Refer to gastroenterologist

Instructions: for each of the patients described below, choose the **single** most appropriate management option from the list above. Each option may be used once, more than once or not at all.

Question 19	A 13 year old girl has pain that occurs during menstruation. She started menstruating one year ago.
Question 20	A 24 year old woman has long-standing symptoms of dysmenorrhoea. She is seeking contraceptive advice.
Question 21	An 18 year old woman has intermittent left iliac fossa pain that is relieved with defaecation. She has not observed a relationship between her symptoms and her menstrual cycle. She had a normal vaginal delivery 6 months ago.

Options for questions 22–24

A	Start oxytocin infusion	F	Call for help
B	Oxytocin intravenous bolus	G	Intramuscular oxytocin and controlled cord traction
C	Intramuscular ergometrine and oxytocin	H	Secure intravenous access
D	Prostaglandins	I	Crossmatch blood
E	Physiological management	J	Intramuscular ergometrine

Instructions: for each of the patients described below, choose the **single** most appropriate management option from the list above. Each option may be used once, more than once or not at all.

Question 22	A 34 year old woman delivered 40 minutes ago. She has opted for active management of the third stage of labour.
Question 23	A 26 year old woman delivered one hour ago. She has opted for physiological management of the third stage of labour.
Question 24	A 30 year old multigravida collapses after delivery. Major postpartum haemorrhage is suspected.

Options for questions 25–27

A	1:20	F	>1:50
B	1:100	G	1:700
C	1:1500	H	1:800
D	1:650	I	1:2000
E	1:200	J	1:400

Instructions: for each of the situations described below, choose the **single** most appropriate risk from the list above. Each option may be used once, more than once or not at all.

Question 25	The risk of having a baby with Down syndrome at the age of 20 years.
Question 26	The risk of having a baby with Down syndrome at the age of 40 years.
Question 27	The risk of having a baby with Edward syndrome in the first trimester.

Options for questions 28–30

A	Combined oral contraceptive pill	F	Ulipristal
B	Levonorgestrel	G	Intrauterine device insertion
C	Depo-Provera only	H	Condom use with nonoxinol '9'
D	Offer a baseline bone scan	I	Depo-Provera and condom use
E	Progestogen-only pill	J	Progestogen subdermal implant

Instructions: for each of the patients described below, choose the **single** most appropriate option from the list above. Each option may be used once, more than once or not at all.

Question 28	A 36 year old woman with AIDS is currently on nevirapine; she would like to choose the most suitable method of contraception.
Question 29	A 36 year old HIV-positive woman on nevirapine is keen to use depot medroxyprogesterone acetate (DMPA).
Question 30	A 20 year old HIV-positive woman had unprotected sexual intercourse 48 hours ago and would like emergency contraception.

Single best answer questions

31 Which one of the following is **not** a risk factor for endometrial carcinoma?

A Obesity.

B Tibolone therapy.

C Women with a history of hereditary non-polyposis colon cancer (HNPCC).

D Multiparity.

E Tamoxifen therapy.

32 Which one of the following statements regarding Klinefelter syndrome is **false**?

A Klinefelter syndrome is the most common sex chromosome disorder.

B Klinefelter syndrome may be associated with an increased risk of breast cancer.

C Klinefelter syndrome may be associated with a decreased risk of osteoporosis.

D Klinefelter syndrome may be associated with learning difficulties.

E Patients with Klinefelter syndrome have a normal life expectancy.

33 Which one of the following statements regarding genital warts is **true**?

A Human papilloma virus (HPV) types 16 and 18 are associated with genital warts.

B Barrier contraception prevents transmission of genital warts.

C The HPV vaccine Cervarix confers protection against genital warts.

D Podophyllotoxin and trichloroacetic acid may be used in the treatment of genital warts.

E Gardasil is a trivalent HPV vaccine.

34 Which one of the following statements regarding hepatitis B is **true**?

A Hepatitis B is not a notifiable illness.

B Hepatitis B is an RNA virus.

C The hepatitis B vaccine should be considered in sex workers.

D 15% of adult patients infected with hepatitis B become carriers.

E Antenatal care does not include hepatitis B testing in the UK.

35 Which one of the following statements regarding ovarian carcinoma is **true**?

A There is a screening programme available for ovarian carcinoma in the UK.

B Hormone replacement therapy taken for more than 5 years may be associated with ovarian cancer.

C Nulliparity is not a risk factor for ovarian carcinoma.

D Ovarian carcinoma presents with early symptoms.

E Hereditary non-polyposis colorectal cancer is not linked with ovarian cancer.

36 Concerning polycystic ovary syndrome (PCOS) which one of the following statements is **false**?

A Women with PCOS should be advised regarding weight control.

B PCOS is associated with sleep apnoea.

C Women with PCOS should be screened for gestational diabetes.

D Women with PCOS may have endometrial hyperplasia.

E Women with PCOS should not be treated with progestogens to induce a withdrawal bleed.

37 Which one of the following statements regarding genital herpes is **true**?

   A Topical antivirals are helpful in the treatment of genital herpes.

   B Genital herpes usually presents with painless ulceration.

   C Antiviral therapy for genital herpes is infrequently given for 5 days.

   D Genital herpes is not caused by herpes simplex virus type 1.

   E Ideally, antiviral therapy for genital herpes should be started within 5 days.

38 Which one of the following statements concerning primary amenorrhoea is **true**?

   A Primary amenorrhoea may apply to girls up to 16 years who have not developed secondary sexual characteristics.

   B Constitutional delay is not a cause of primary amenorrhoea.

   C Turner syndrome may be associated with primary amenorrhoea.

   D Imperforate hymen is not a cause of primary amenorrhoea.

   E Hyperprolactinaemia does not cause primary amenorrhoea.

39 Regarding the HPV vaccine, which one of the following statements is **true**?

   A Cervarix is a quadrivalent HPV vaccine.

   B Cervarix confers protection against genital warts.

   C The first dose is given to all 12–13 year old children.

   D Vaccination may be given during pregnancy.

   E Three doses are required.

40 Concerning vulvovaginal candidiasis which one of the following is **false**?

   A Vulvovaginal candidiasis is associated with pregnancy.

   B Vulvovaginal candidiasis is associated with antibiotic use.

C Diabetes increases the risk of vulvovaginal candidiasis.

D Vulvovaginal candidiasis may present with dysuria.

E Candida albicans is a pathological organism in the vagina.

41 Which one of the following statements regarding breech presentation is **true**?

A Previous breech delivery is not a risk factor for breech presentation.

B Breech babies do not require careful neonatal hip examination.

C Congenital malformations do not increase the risk of breech presentation.

D Low birth weight is associated with breech presentation.

E Singleton pregnancies have an increased rate of breech presentation.

42 Regarding gestational diabetes which one of the following statements is **true**?

A Women diagnosed with gestational diabetes should be offered an oral glucose tolerance test at the 6-week postnatal check.

B BMI ≥28 kg/m² is a risk factor for screening for gestational diabetes.

C A previously macrosomic baby weighing >3.5 kg is a risk factor for screening for gestational diabetes.

D If there is no previous history of gestational diabetes, an oral glucose tolerance test may be done at 16–18 weeks if there are risk factors for gestational diabetes.

E If there is no previous history of gestational diabetes an oral glucose tolerance test may be done at 24–28 weeks if there are risk factors for gestational diabetes.

43 Which one of the following statements is **false**?

A Valproate therapy should not be prescribed to women of child-bearing age routinely.

B Women taking antipsychotics may have raised prolactin levels resulting in subfertility.

C Olanzepine may be associated with gestational diabetes.

D Puerperal psychosis occurs in approximately 1 in 10 000 mothers.

E Postnatal depression usually develops in the first month after childbirth.

44 Which one of the following statements regarding Turner syndrome is **true**?

A Turner syndrome is not associated with gonadal dysgenesis.

B Turner syndrome is associated with tall stature.

C Turner syndrome cannot arise as a result of mosaicism.

D Neonatal lymphoedema of the hands and feet is not a feature of Turner syndrome.

E Turner syndrome is associated with coarctation of the aorta.

45 With regard to child maltreatment which one of the following statements is **false**?

A Child maltreatment may be suspected in a child where there is bruising (not caused by a medical condition) in a child who is not independently mobile.

B Child maltreatment may be suspected in a child with fractures of different ages if there is no medical condition that predisposes to fragile bones.

C Retinal haemorrhages may be a feature of child maltreatment in the absence of accidental trauma.

D Gonorrhoea in a 12 year old girl is unlikely to represent child maltreatment.

E Child maltreatment may be suspected in a child where there is a torn frenulum of the upper lip.

46 Which one of the following WHO reference values for semen analysis is **correct**?

A   Volume ≥1 ml.

B   Motility ≥70%.

C   Total sperm number ≥40 x10^6 spermatozoa per ejaculate.

D   Sperm concentration ≥10 x10^6 per ml.

E   Liquefaction time within 30 minutes.

47 Which one of the following statements concerning secondary amenorrhoea is **false**?

A   Rapid weight loss may result in secondary amenorrhoea.

B   Excessive physical exercise may result in secondary amenorrhoea.

C   Phenothiazines may cause secondary amenorrhoea.

D   Depot medroxyprogesterone acetate may cause secondary amenorrhoea.

E   Sheehan syndrome does not cause secondary amenorrhoea.

48 Which one of the following statements regarding syphilis is **true**?

A   Syphilis is caused by the protozoan *Treponema pallidum*.

B   Secondary syphilis typically presents with a painless genital ulcer.

C   The incubation period may be up to 30 days.

D   Primary syphilis may present with a widespread skin rash.

E   Tertiary syphilis may develop 3 years after initial infection.

Multiple choice questions

For each of these multiple choice questions, you must indicate which of the statements are true and which are false.

49 Concerning female barrier contraception

A   Diaphragm or caps used with spermicide may be up to 90% effective.

B   The diaphragm or cap should be left *in situ* for 3 hours after sexual intercourse.

C   Additional spermicide should be used if the diaphragm or cervical cap has been left *in situ* for more than 1 hour prior to sexual intercourse.

D   The diaphragm or cap may need to be re-fitted after a woman has been pregnant.

E   The diaphragm or cap provides protection against HIV transmission.

50 Concerning cervical cancer and screening

A   Cervical screening is not recommended after the age of 64 years.

B   Human papilloma viruses 6 and 11 are associated with cervical cancers.

C   Genital warts increase the risk of cervical cancer.

D   Having multiple sexual partners increases the risk of cervical cancer.

E   HIV status may influence the risk of developing cervical cancer.

51 Regarding asthma and pregnancy

A   Asthma may worsen in one-third of women during pregnancy.

B   Leukotriene antagonists should be stopped during pregnancy.

C   If there is an acute severe asthma attack during pregnancy, intermittent fetal monitoring is recommended.

D   Acute asthma is rare during labour.

E   Breastfeeding is not recommended for mothers with asthma.

52 Regarding puerperal pyrexia

A Puerperal pyrexia may be diagnosed in women up to 28 days postpartum.

B Puerperal pyrexia may be diagnosed in women up to 30 days postpartum.

C In puerperal pyrexia the lower legs should be examined.

D In puerperal pyrexia an assessment of perineal wounds is not appropriate.

E In puerperal pyrexia a history of urinary catheterisation should be sought.

53 Lichen sclerosus:

A Is seen more commonly in men than in women.

B In a woman may cause superficial dyspareunia.

C Is not associated with an increased risk of vulval cancer.

D Does not cause itching.

E Often responds to a strong topical steroid preparation.

54 Regarding ectopic pregnancy

A There is a decreased risk of ectopic pregnancy in women with a previous history of tubal surgery.

B Pelvic inflammatory disease increases the risk of ectopic pregnancy.

C Endometriosis increases the risk of ectopic pregnancy.

D Infertility treatments may increase the risk of ectopic pregnancy.

E If pregnancy should result from a contraceptive failure with the progestogen-only pill, there is a decreased risk of ectopic pregnancy when compared with other methods of contraception.

55 Regarding the cervix

A The lower two-thirds of the cervix has stratified squamous epithelium.

B An ectropion is caused when columnar epithelium extends through the internal os.

C Cervical ectopy is associated with the menopause.

D Cervical ectopy may be associated with the oral contraceptive pill.

E Nabothian cysts usually present with bleeding.

56 Concerning acute appendicitis and pregnancy

A Acute appendicitis is the most common general surgical condition during pregnancy.

B Acute appendicitis during the third trimester typically presents with right lower quadrant pain.

C Acute appendicitis is not associated with an increased risk of preterm labour.

D Perforation of the appendix is more likely in the first trimester.

E There is an increased risk of appendicitis during pregnancy.

57 Regarding heroin use and pregnancy

A Heroin use during pregnancy does not increase the risk of intrauterine growth restriction.

B Heroin use during pregnancy does not increase the risk of premature labour.

C Heroin use during pregnancy may cause neonatal withdrawal syndrome.

D Methadone maintenance therapy is preferable to heroin use during pregnancy.

E Heroin users may be at an increased risk of blood-borne infection.

58 Concerning advancing maternal age and pregnancy

A There is an increased rate of miscarriage with increased maternal age.

B Advancing maternal age does not increase the risk of gestational diabetes.

C Advancing maternal age is not linked to an increase in Caesarean section rate.

D There is an increased rate of instrumental delivery with increased maternal age.

E Hypertensive disorders occur more commonly with advanced maternal age.

59 Regarding inflammatory bowel disease (IBD) and pregnancy

A Women with IBD should be given pre-conceptual advice about folic acid.

B Azathioprine may be used during pregnancy to control IBD.

C Methotrexate should be stopped for at least 2 months in a woman prior to attempting to conceive.

D Methotrexate should be stopped for at least 3 months in a man prior to attempting to conceive.

E Women with severe IBD have an increased risk of preterm delivery.

60 Regarding antepartum haemorrhage (APH)

A Rhesus-negative women with APH do not need to be given anti-D immunoglobulin.

B APH is often defined as bleeding after the 28th week of pregnancy.

C Placenta praevia typically causes recurrent painful bleeding.

D Vaginal examination may safely be carried out in suspected APH.

E APH is more common in primiparous women.

61 Concerning postpartum contraception

A The combined oral contraceptive pill may be started 2 weeks after birth if not breastfeeding.

B The progesterone-only pill may be started 1 week postpartum.

C Depot medroxyprogesterone acetate may be given within 5 days postpartum if not breastfeeding.

D Depot medroxyprogesterone acetate may be given within 4 weeks postpartum if breastfeeding.

E The subdermal implant Nexplanon may be given 2 weeks after delivery.

62 Regarding hepatitis C and pregnancy

A Vertical transmission of hepatitis C occurs in 70% of cases.

B There is an increased risk of vertical transmission of hepatitis C if there is co-infection with HIV.

C Antenatal hepatitis C screening is carried out in the UK.

D Screening for hepatitis C may be offered to women who are HIV positive.

E Caesarean section significantly reduces vertical transmission of hepatitis C.

63 Concerning toxoplasmosis and pregnancy

A Pregnant women should avoid contact with cat litter to reduce the risk of transmission of toxoplasmosis.

B Toxoplasmosis is caused by a bacterium.

C Fetal infection most commonly occurs in the first trimester.

D Congenital toxoplasmosis is more severe if infection occurs in the third trimester.

E Hydrocephalus may be caused by toxoplasmosis.

64 Concerning perineal tears

A A second degree tear involves injury to the perineal muscles.

B A third degree tear refers to perineal injury with disruption of the anal sphincter muscles and breach of the rectal mucosa.

C A fourth degree tear does not involve the anal sphincter muscles.

D A fourth degree tear breaches the rectal mucosa.

E In a second degree tear the anal sphincter is disrupted.

65 Concerning sexually transmitted infections and antibiotics

A Syphilis cannot be treated with benzathine benzylpenicillin.

B Uncomplicated gonorrhoea may be treated with ciprofloxacin.

C Ceftriaxone is not used to treat pharyngeal gonorrhoea infection.

D Uncomplicated chlamydia may be treated with a single dose of doxycycline.

E Pelvic inflammatory disease should be treated for at least 10 days.

66 Regarding exomphalos and gastroschisis

A Gastroschisis is usually associated with other congenital defects.

B Both conditions may be associated with reduced maternal serum alpha-fetoprotein levels.

C Exomphalos usually occurs on the right side of the umbilical cord.

D In exomphalos the abdominal contents are covered by a membrane.

E Gastroschisis usually occurs to the left side of umbilical cord.

67 Domestic violence:

A In the family increases the risk of physical abuse in children.

B Infrequently occurs during pregnancy.

C   In pregnancy is not associated with an increased risk of miscarriage.

D   Typically stops after a violent relationship has ended.

E   May have alcohol misuse as a contributory factor.

68   Clomifene:

A   Activates oestrogen receptors in the hypothalamus.

B   Does not cause hot flushes.

C   May be given continuously.

D   Therapy should be withdrawn if there is visual disturbance.

E   Therapy does not cause ovarian hyperstimulation.

69   Regarding Patau syndrome

A   Patau syndrome is caused by trisomy 18.

B   There is an increased risk of Patau syndrome with advancing maternal age.

C   Facial clefting is not a feature of Patau syndrome.

D   Holoprosencephaly is a feature of Patau syndrome.

E   Patau syndrome commonly causes cardiac defects.

70   Concerning meconium:

A   Meconium aspiration does not cause surfactant dysfunction.

B   Meconium aspiration usually occurs as a result of fetal hypoxia.

C   There is an increased risk of passage of meconium in pre-eclampsia.

D   Cocaine use decreases the risk of passage of meconium.

E   There is an increased risk of passage of meconium in oligohydramnios.

71 Regarding Apgar score

A   The Apgar score is used to assess a baby at 2 and 10 minutes post-delivery.

B   The maximum Apgar score is 12.

C   The Apgar score does not take into account muscle tone.

D   The Apgar score takes into account respiratory effort.

E   The colour of the baby is relevant in the Apgar score.

72 Regarding air travel and pregnancy

A   There is not an increased risk of venous thromboembolism associated with air travel during pregnancy.

B   It is recommended that air travel is avoided in uncomplicated singleton pregnancies at the end of 34 weeks of gestation.

C   It is recommended that air travel is avoided in uncomplicated multiple pregnancies at 28 weeks of gestation.

D   It is recommended that air travel is avoided in uncomplicated multiple pregnancies at 32 weeks of gestation.

E   Fetal PaO_2 is compromised at cabin altitude.

73 Regarding the CA125 protein marker

A   CA125 may be used to monitor patients for relapse in ovarian cancer.

B   Pregnancy does not cause an elevated CA125 level.

C   Pelvic inflammatory disease does not cause an elevated CA125 level.

D   Endometriosis may cause an elevated CA125 level.

E   CA125 is used to screen for ovarian cancer in the UK.

74 Concerning statistics

A   Sensitivity is obtained by calculating the proportion of people who have a positive test result who actually have the disease.

B   Specificity is the proportion of people who have a disease but test negative for the condition.

C   A false negative is where the disease is absent and the test is positive.

D   A false positive is where the disease is present and the test is negative.

E   A false positive is where the disease is absent and the test is positive.

75 Regarding management of pre-eclampsia

A   Korotkoff phase 3 is the appropriate measurement of diastolic blood pressure.

B   Systolic blood pressure decreases in the 2nd trimester of pregnancy.

C   Pregnancy-induced hypertension is associated with proteinuria.

D   Diagnosis may include visual symptoms.

E   At the postnatal check an assessment of blood pressure and proteinuria should be made.

76 Ulipristal:

A   Is not as effective as levonorgestrel in preventing pregnancy.

B   Is more effective in preventing pregnancy than an intrauterine device.

C   May only be used within 72 hours of unprotected sexual intercourse.

D   May be bought over the counter in selected pharmacies.

E   May require another dose if a woman vomits within 5 hours of taking it.

77 Regarding risks of abdominal hysterectomy

A The ureter may be damaged during abdominal hysterectomy.

B Blood loss requiring blood transfusion rarely occurs after abdominal hysterectomy.

C There is a high risk of pelvic abscess formation after routine abdominal hysterectomy.

D There is a high risk of bowel perforation during routine abdominal hysterectomy.

E Venous thromboembolism prophylaxis should be considered pre-operatively.

78 Concerning Fraser guidelines

A Contraceptive advice or treatment may be given to a 15 year old girl who has capacity and cannot be persuaded to inform her parents.

B Contraceptive advice or treatment may be given to a 15 year old girl who has capacity and is likely to have sexual intercourse.

C Contraceptive advice or treatment may be given to a 14 year old girl who has capacity, if it is in her best interest.

D Teenagers aged less than 14 years are not considered to have capacity to consent to sexual activity.

E Confidentiality may be upheld in all circumstances.

79 Bacterial vaginosis (BV):

A Is more common in sexually active women.

B Is a sexually transmitted infection.

C May cause a frothy yellow discharge.

D Is associated with a decrease in pH in the vagina.

E Is not associated with an increased risk of preterm birth.

80 Regarding alternatives to hormone replacement therapy

A   The vasomotor symptoms of the menopause may be triggered by alcohol.

B   Selective serotonin re-uptake inhibitors are licensed for the treatment of menopausal symptoms.

C   Clonidine is not licensed for the treatment of vasomotor symptoms of the menopause.

D   The vasomotor symptoms of the menopause may be triggered by caffeine.

E   There is good evidence that black cohosh reduces the vasomotor symptoms of the menopause.

81 Concerning medroxyprogesterone (Depo-Provera)

A   Medroxyprogesterone is not associated with an irregular bleeding pattern.

B   There is a delayed return of fertility when medroxyprogesterone is discontinued.

C   It is given within the first 10 days of a cycle.

D   If the interval is 12 weeks and 2 days between injections, pregnancy should be excluded.

E   In women who are breastfeeding the injection should be delayed until 4 weeks postpartum.

82 Pruritic Urticated Papules and Plaques of Pregnancy (PUPPP):

A   Usually arises in the 2nd trimester.

B   Does not improve after delivery.

C   Typically appears initially on abdominal striae.

D   Does not affect the limbs.

E   Shows a positive result on direct immunofluorescence.

83 Concerning respiratory distress syndrome

A   There is an increased risk of respiratory distress syndrome with Caesarean section.

B   There is a decreased risk of respiratory distress syndrome with premature delivery.

C   Maternal diabetes is not associated with neonatal respiratory distress syndrome.

D   Meconium aspiration is not associated with neonatal respiratory distress syndrome.

E   The risk of neonatal respiratory distress syndrome may be reduced by administration of antenatal corticosteroids.

84 Regarding malaria and pregnancy

A   Malaria during pregnancy is not associated with an increased rate of miscarriage.

B   Malaria during pregnancy is not associated with an increased rate of fetal growth restriction.

C   A travel history should be sought in a pregnant woman presenting with pyrexia of unknown origin.

D   Hyperglycaemia is a maternal complication of malaria during pregnancy.

E   Pulmonary oedema is not a maternal complication of malaria during pregnancy.

85 Regarding natural family planning

A   Sexual intercourse should be avoided for 10 days prior to ovulation.

B   Sexual intercourse should be avoided for 1–2 days after ovulation.

C   Ovulation may be predicted by a slight decrease in body temperature.

D   Ovulation may be predicted by detecting changes in vaginal secretions.

E   Natural family planning may be difficult if a woman has irregular periods.

86 Concerning vitamin K deficiency bleeding (VKDB):

A Early VKDB occurs within 48 hours of birth.

B Babies that are breastfed are at decreased risk of this condition when compared with formula-fed babies.

C Coeliac disease is not a risk factor for VKDB.

D It is recommended that all newborn babies receive vitamin K to prevent VKDB.

E Two oral doses of phytomenadione are given to exclusively breastfed babies to prevent VKDB.

87 With regard to ovarian hyperstimulation syndrome (OHSS)

A Mild OHSS affects up to 5% of *in vitro* fertilisation cycles.

B Symptoms may arise up to 5 days prior to egg harvesting.

C Severe OHSS may cause ascites.

D There is an increased risk of OHSS with advanced maternal age.

E There is a decreased risk of OHSS with polycystic ovary disease.

88 Concerning Potter syndrome

A Potter syndrome is caused by polyhydramnios.

B Posterior urethral valves are not a risk factor for Potter syndrome.

C A recessed chin and prominent epicanthal folds may be features of Potter syndrome.

D Polycystic kidney disease is not a risk factor for Potter syndrome.

E There may be respiratory distress at birth.

Answers and explanations for exam paper 3

1. Answer E Intravenous iron infusion

Women are screened for anaemia at the booking visit and at 28 weeks. Anaemia is confirmed by Hb <11 g/dl at the booking visit. Oral iron should be used first-line for iron-deficiency anaemia. Parenteral iron may be considered if oral iron is not tolerated.

2. Answer H Haemoglobin electrophoresis

If haemoglobin is <10.5 g/dl antenatally, haemoglobinopathy should be considered. If haemoglobinopathy is excluded, haematinic deficiency should be considered.

3. Answer J Iron deficiency anaemia

Anaemia in pregnancy may be the result of haemodilution due to the increase in plasma volume and the needs of the growing fetus; it is commonly iron-deficiency anaemia. Women are screened for anaemia at the booking visit and at 28 weeks.

4. Answer A Anti-D is not recommended

In Rhesus-negative women who have a Rhesus-positive fetus, fetomaternal haemorrhage is associated with the risk of developing anti-D antibodies. Anti-D should be given following a threatened miscarriage after 12 weeks of gestation to Rhesus-negative women that have not been sensitised. There is a paucity of evidence to suggest that bleeding before this time causes sensitisation, therefore routine anti-D is not recommended. The use of anti-D may be considered if there is heavy bleeding or abdominal pain associated with a threatened miscarriage. In this scenario there is minimal vaginal spotting that has stopped therefore routine anti-D is not recommended.

5. Answer F Anti-D is recommended

All Rhesus D-negative women who give birth to a Rhesus-positive baby should be offered anti-D 72 hours after delivery. Sensitisation to the Rhesus antigen may occur after chorionic villus biopsy and external cephalic version. For routine antenatal prophylaxis NICE (2008; *Pregnancy (rhesus negative women) – routine anti-D (review)*, TA156) recommends that two doses of anti-D immunoglobulin should be given at 28 weeks and at 34 weeks of gestation; alternatively a single dose may be given between 28 and 30 weeks of gestation (*BNF*).

6. Answer E Check middle cerebral artery peak systolic velocity

This scenario is suggestive of haemolytic disease of the newborn; antenatal ultrasound has not indicated signs of fetal hydrops. Fetal anaemia may be assessed by Doppler imaging of the middle cerebral artery in the first instance. Fetal blood sampling may be required.

7. Answer C Mid-stream urine for culture and microscopy

Risks of abdominal hysterectomy include damage to the bladder and/or the ureter, blood loss requiring blood transfusion, wound infection, pain, urinary tract infection and ovarian failure. In this scenario a urinary tract infection should be excluded.

8. Answer E Diagnostic laparoscopy

Endometriosis is a condition in which hormonally responsive endometrial tissue is found outside the uterus. Endometriosis is therefore generally confined to women in their reproductive age. Women may report dyspareunia; this is more likely to be a feature of severe disease. Moreover this may be associated with an immobile fixed retroverted uterus. Dysmenorrhoea, chronic pelvic pain and infertility may also be caused by endometriosis. In this scenario, diagnostic laparoscopy should be carried out to ascertain the diagnosis.

9. Answer B Hormone replacement therapy

In this scenario, menopausal symptoms may be managed with HRT after an informed discussion with the patient. Hysterectomy with or without oophorectomy may result in premature menopause. A hormonal profile is not usually necessary to diagnose the menopause, but if there is diagnostic doubt a hormonal profile may be helpful.

10. Answer H Antibiotics and continue breastfeeding

Postpartum causes of pyrexia include urinary tract and genital tract infections, mastitis, wound infection and deep vein thrombosis. Breast infections are commonly caused by *Staphylococcus aureus*; breastfeeding may continue whilst receiving appropriate antibiotics for mastitis.

11. Answer A Risk greater than 1 in 150

From 11 to 13^{+6} weeks of gestation, the combined test may be performed for screening for Down syndrome. Diagnostic testing may be offered to a woman as a result of 1st trimester screening if the risk is greater than 1 in 150.

12. Answer **G** Transvaginal scan

Women presenting with postmenopausal bleeding and who are not taking HRT, and those on tamoxifen with postmenopausal bleeding, should be referred urgently under the 2 week wait rule for further investigation. Women with persistent or unexplained postmenopausal bleeding after stopping HRT for 6 weeks should be referred urgently under the 2 week wait rule for further investigation. In this scenario transvaginal ultrasound to assess endometrial thickness is the most appropriate option.

13. Answer **G** Endometrial cancer

Postmenopausal bleeding may be a symptom of endometrial cancer. The following are risk factors for endometrial carcinoma: obesity, tibolone therapy, tamoxifen therapy, nulliparity and women with a history of hereditary non-polyposis colon cancer (HNPCC). Women presenting with postmenopausal bleeding who are taking tamoxifen should be referred urgently under the 2 week wait rule for further investigation.

14. Answer **C** Atrophic endometrium

Transvaginal ultrasound to assess endometrial thickness may be carried out as a first-line investigation in postmenopausal bleeding. If the endometrium is thicker than expected in a postmenopausal woman, hysteroscopy and biopsy should be considered. In this scenario an endometrial thickness of less than 4 mm is reassuring. According to the NHS Cervical Screening Programme, all women between the ages of 25 and 64 are eligible for cervical screening.

15. Answer **B** Cervical polyp

In this scenario a recent cervical smear was normal, therefore a cervical polyp represents the most likely option. Cervical polyps are usually asymptomatic but may present with postcoital and intermenstrual bleeding.

16. Answer **G** Laparotomy

An ectopic pregnancy is one that occurs at any other site apart from the endometrium. The majority of ectopic pregnancies occur in the Fallopian tubes. Management of ectopic pregnancy may involve salpingectomy or salpingostomy which may be performed both by laparoscopy or laparotomy. In a haemodynamically unstable patient, emergency laparotomy is the most appropriate option

17. Answer **A** Expectant management

Expectant management may be appropriate for women with minimal symptoms and a pregnancy of unknown location. In a pregnancy of unknown location, β-hCG is less than 1000 IU/l and there is no visible pregnancy seen on transvaginal ultrasound. In women managed expectantly serial β-hCG levels should be carried out.

18. Answer **D** Laparoscopic salpingectomy

Medical management is contraindicated in this scenario as cardiac activity in an ectopic pregnancy has been visualised. Laparoscopic salpingectomy is the treatment of choice in a haemodynamically stable patient. If the Fallopian tube is irreparably damaged or diseased, salpingectomy is the preferred procedure as there is a significant risk of recurrence of ectopic pregnancy in a diseased tube with salpingostomy.

19. Answer **F** Antiprostaglandins

Primary dysmenorrhoea may result from prostaglandin and leukotriene release causing vasoconstriction of the uterine vessels as well as uterine contractions. Symptoms often coincide with the development of ovulatory cycles in primary dysmenorrhoea. Secondary dysmenorrhoea may be due to fibroids, pelvic inflammatory disease and endometriosis. In this scenario, a trial of non-steroidal anti-inflammatory drugs would be appropriate. This would result in the inhibition of cyclo-oxygenase thereby reducing prostaglandin production. If this was ineffective the combined oral contraceptive pill may be considered.

20. Answer **D** Combined oral contraceptive pill

Combined oral contraceptives may be used to treat dysmenorrhoea, premenstrual tension and menorrhagia. Combined oral contraceptive use may be associated with less symptomatic fibroids and functional ovarian cysts.

21. Answer **I** Irritable bowel syndrome

Irritable bowel syndrome is a diagnosis of exclusion. The diagnosis may be considered in those with abdominal pain relieved by defaecation or associated with altered bowel frequency. Other symptoms include straining, incomplete evacuation, abdominal bloating and symptoms associated with eating.

22. Answer **H** Secure intravenous access

Intravenous access should be secured if there is a delay in the third stage of greater than 30 minutes after birth with active management (*NICE*, 2008; *Intrapartum care*, CG55). Active management involves giving intramuscular oxytocin and early cord clamping with controlled cord traction. Oxytocin may then be given into the umbilical vein after intravenous access is secured and the proximal cord has been clamped.

23. Answer G Intramuscular oxytocin and controlled cord traction

Physiological management refers to a third stage where there is delivery by maternal effort. Oxytocin, cord clamping and cord traction are not employed. If there is a delay in the third stage of greater than 1 hour after birth with physiological management, active management is recommended. Active management involves giving intramuscular oxytocin and early cord clamping with controlled cord traction.

24. Answer F Call for help

Multiple pregnancy is a risk factor for postpartum haemorrhage. In this scenario it is important to call for help. Major postpartum haemorrhage should be managed according to resuscitation principles. The airway, breathing and circulation should be assessed and intravenous access obtained.

25. Answer C 1:1500

The underlying genetic basis for Down syndrome is trisomy 21 in most cases; it may also arise as a result of translocations and mosaicism. Maternal age is a risk factor, for example the risk may be approximately 1:1500 at 20 years, 1:400 at 35 years, 1:100 at 40 years and 1:30 at 45 years. Furthermore the risk is increased if there has been a previously affected pregnancy.

26. Answer B 1:100

The underlying genetic basis for Down syndrome is trisomy 21 in most cases; it may also arise as a result of translocations and mosaicism. Maternal age is a risk factor, for example the risk may be approximately 1:1500 at 20 years, 1:400 at 35 years, 1:100 at 40 years and 1:30 at 45 years. Furthermore the risk is increased if there has been a previously affected pregnancy.

27. Answer J 1:400

Edward syndrome occurs as a result of trisomy 18. The incidence of trisomy 18 is 1:400 at first trimester screening. However, it only affects 1 in 6000 live births because the majority of affected fetuses do not survive.

28. Answer I Depo-Provera and condom use

In HIV-positive women not taking antiretroviral therapy, consideration may be given to all contraceptive methods available. In addition condom use should be encouraged to reduce the risk of HIV transmission. The efficacy of the combined oral contraceptive pill, the progestogen-only pill and the progestogen-only subdermal implant may be reduced with antiretroviral drugs; therefore additional contraceptive cover is required. In women taking antiretroviral therapy, DMPA and intrauterine devices may be appropriate. In this scenario use of Depo-Provera and encouraging condom use represents the best option. Spermicidal contraceptives such as nonoxinol '9' are unsuitable in HIV-positive individuals. In this scenario there is evidence of immunosuppression and therefore intrauterine device insertion is contraindicated.

29. Answer D Offer a baseline bone scan

DMPA users may benefit from having a baseline bone density scan as both HIV and some antiretrovirals may reduce bone mineral density.

30. Answer G Intrauterine device insertion

In HIV-positive women on antiretroviral therapy, the emergency intrauterine device is the most effective method when compared with emergency hormonal contraception. If emergency hormonal contraception is used an increased dose should be taken in those taking enzyme-inducing drugs.

31. Answer D

The following are risk factors for endometrial carcinoma: obesity, tibolone therapy, tamoxifen therapy, nulliparity and women with a history of hereditary non-polyposis colon cancer (HNPCC).

32. Answer C

Klinefelter syndrome is the most common sex chromosome disorder; those affected have an additional X chromosome. Features of Klinefelter syndrome include loss of libido, gynaecomastia, impaired spermatogenesis, hypogonadism, osteoporosis and an increased risk of breast cancer. In childhood, the condition may present with delayed speech or learning difficulties.

33. Answer D

Genital warts are caused by different types of the human papilloma virus (HPV); they usually arise from direct skin contact during sexual intercourse. HPV types 6 and 11 are associated with genital warts. They may arise several months after infection. Barrier contraception may reduce the risk of HPV transmission. Genital warts may cause itching, bleeding or pain. Treatment options may include cryotherapy, podophyllotoxin, trichloroacetic acid, excision or diathermy. The HPV vaccine Gardasil is effective against HPV types 6, 11, 16 and 18.

34. Answer C

Hepatitis B is a notifiable disease in the UK that is also screened for antenatally. It is caused by the hepatits B virus which is a DNA virus. It may be transmitted sexually, through blood contact and perinatally. It may present as an acute infection or with jaundice, hepatitis B surface antigen tests may be positive

1–6 months after exposure. Five per cent or fewer of adult patients infected with hepatitis B develop chronic hepatitis infection. This group are hepatitis B carriers and are hepatitis B surface antigen-positive. Hepatitis B carriers may develop liver cirrhosis and have an increased risk of developing hepatocellular carcinoma. The hepatitis B vaccine should be considered in sex workers.

35. Answer B

Ovarian carcinoma is associated with more than 5 years of HRT, nulliparity and a family history of breast and ovarian cancer. It usually presents at an advanced stage with symptoms such as abdominal distension, weight loss and dyspepsia; it may present with a pelvic or abdominal mass. There is no UK screening programme for ovarian carcinoma. Hereditary non-polyposis colorectal cancer may be associated with ovarian and endometrial cancers.

36. Answer E

Polycystic ovary syndrome is associated with obstructive sleep apnoea, impaired glucose tolerance and type 2 diabetes. Women with PCOS should be advised regarding weight control. Oligomenorrhoea or amenorrhoea in women with PCOS may predispose to endometrial hyperplasia and possibly carcinoma. The RCOG recommends treatment with progestogens to induce a withdrawal bleed at least every 3–4 months (*RCOG*, 2007; *Green-top Guideline 33: Long-term consequences of polycystic ovary syndrome*).

37. Answer E

Genital herpes may be caused by herpes simplex viruses types 1 and 2, however, type 2 is usually associated with genital infection. It usually presents with multiple painful ulcers. It is usually managed with oral treatment which should be started as soon as possible, ideally within 5 days. Antiviral therapy may reduce the severity and duration of an episode of genital herpes. It is usually given for 5 days, but the course may be extended if new lesions appear during treatment, or if the patient is immunocompromised.

38. Answer C

Primary amenorrhoea may apply to girls up to 14 years who have not developed secondary sexual characteristics or to girls up to 16 years with normal secondary sexual characteristics. Primary amenorrhoea may be due to constitutional delay, imperforate hymen, or uterine or vaginal malformations. Hypothalamic–pituitary axis failure may result in the absence of secondary sexual characteristics; causes include hyperprolactinaemia and ovarian dysgenesis in Turner syndrome.

39. Answer E

The HPV vaccine is available as the bivalent vaccine Cervarix or as the quadrivalent vaccine Gardasil. Cervarix is licensed for use in females for the prevention of cervical cancer and other pre-cancerous lesions caused by HPV types 16 and 18. Additionally Gardasil confers protection against HPV 6 and 11 and therefore may prevent genital warts. Both vaccinations are licensed for use in females; the national programme is aimed at girls aged 12–13 years. The second and third doses are given at 1–2 months and 6 months after the initial dose. It is recommended that the vaccinations are postponed until completion of pregnancy; however, the vaccines are not known to be harmful in pregnancy.

40. Answer E

Vulvovaginal candidiasis is commonly caused by *Candida albicans*. *C. albicans* is a commensal organism found in the vagina. Vulvovaginal candidiasis is associated with pregnancy, diabetes and treatment with broad-spectrum antibiotics. It may present with itching, white discharge and dysuria.

41. Answer D

With increased gestation there is less likelihood of breech position. Breech presentation may be associated with multiple pregnancy, low birth weight, congenital malformation, previous breech delivery, placenta praevia, uterine anomalies and developmental dysplasia of the hip.

42. Answer E

Women diagnosed with gestational diabetes should be offered lifestyle advice and a fasting plasma glucose level at the 6 week postnatal check. The following are risk factors for the screening for gestational diabetes: BMI >30 kg/m², a previously macrosomic baby weighing ≥4.5 kg, a first degree relative with diabetes, and family history with a high prevalence of diabetes. If there is no previous history of gestational diabetes, an oral glucose tolerance test may be done at 24–28 weeks if there are risk factors for gestational diabetes. If there is a previous history of gestational diabetes, an oral glucose tolerance test may be done at 16–18 weeks (*NICE*, 2008; *Diabetes in pregnancy*, CG63).

43. Answer D

Valproate therapy should not be prescribed to women of child-bearing age routinely due to the increased risk of fetal neural tube defects. Women taking antipsychotics such as amisulpiride and risperidone may have raised prolactin levels resulting in subfertility. Olanzepine may be associated with weight gain and gestational diabetes (*NICE*, 2007; *Antenatal and postnatal mental health*, CG45). Puerperal psychosis occurs in approximately 1 in 1000 mothers. Postnatal depression usually develops in the first month after childbirth; 'baby blues' occurs in the first few days postpartum.

44. Answer E

Turner syndrome is the most common sex chromosome abnormality in females; it may be caused by the absence of one X chromosome (45,X) or may result from mosaicism (for example: 45,X/46,XX). Features include short stature, lymphoedema of the hands and feet at birth, gonadal dysgenesis, high palate, widely spaced nipples, wide carrying angle and a webbed neck. Cardiovascular features include an increased risk of coarctation of the aorta and bicuspid aortic valve.

45. Answer D

If there is no clear evidence of vertical transmission, a sexually transmitted infection in a child less than 13 years is likely to represent child maltreatment. Sex with a child under 13 years is unlawful (*NICE*, 2009; *When to suspect child maltreatment*, CG68). Risk factors for child maltreatment include a previous history of child abuse in the family, domestic violence, substance misuse and social deprivation.

46. Answer C

WHO reference values for semen analysis include: volume ≥ 2 ml, liquefaction time within 60 minutes, pH ≥ 7.2, sperm concentration $\geq 20 \times 10^6$ per ml, total sperm number $\geq 40 \times 10^6$ spermatozoa per ejaculate, and motility $\geq 50\%$. According to NICE (2004; *Infertility*, CG11), screening for anti-sperm antibodies is not required.

47. Answer E

Secondary amenorrhoea may be caused by pregnancy, premature ovarian failure, rapid weight loss, excessive physical exercise, hyperprolactinaemia (phenothiazines may cause hyperprolactinaemia), Sheehan syndrome, PCOS, Nexplanon and depot medroxyprogesterone acetate (DMPA).

48. Answer E

Syphilis is a sexually transmitted bacterial infection caused by *Treponema pallidum;* recently there has been an increase in rates of syphilis amongst men who have sex with men. In the primary phase syphilis may be undetected or may present as a painless genital ulcer. There is an incubation period of up to 90 days. After 3 weeks, a widespread skin rash may develop as well as a febrile illness. Tertiary syphilis may develop 3 years or more after initial infection.

49. Answer FFFTF

Women using the diaphragm or cervical caps should be advised to attend for contraceptive review if they have lost or gained weight of more than 3 kg or they have been pregnant as they may need re-fitting. Diaphragm or caps used with spermicide may be up to 96% effective if there is reliable use. Additional spermicide should be used if the diaphragm or cervical cap has been left *in situ* for more than 3 hours prior to sexual intercourse. Following intercourse, the diaphragm or cap should be left *in situ* for 6 hours. These methods may not be effective in preventing HIV transmission.

50. Answer **FFFTT**

Women at the upper age limit of cervical screening may be screened if they have not been screened previously. HPV 16 and 18 are associated with cervical cancer, HPV 6 and 11 are linked to genital warts. A history of multiple sexual partners is associated with an increased risk of exposure to HPV, which in turn may increase the risk of cervical cancer. Immunosuppression increases the risk of cervical cancer.

51. Answer **TFFTF**

During pregnancy, asthma may worsen in one-third of women; it may improve in one-third and may remain stable in one-third. The risk of adverse maternal and fetal outcomes may be reduced by good asthma control during pregnancy (*British Thoracic Society*, 2009; *British Guidelines on the Management of Asthma*). Short-acting β_2-agonists may be used as normal during pregnancy. Leukotriene antagonists may be continued during pregnancy if asthma control is best achieved this way. Drug treatment for an acute asthma attack is the same during pregnancy as it is for the non-pregnant patient. If there is an acute severe asthma attack during pregnancy, continuous fetal monitoring is recommended. Acute asthma is rare during labour. Breastfeeding is recommended for mothers with asthma.

52. Answer **FFTFT**

Puerperal pyrexia is the presence of fever $\geq 38°C$ in a woman who is up to 14 days postpartum. Postpartum causes of pyrexia include urinary and genital tract infections, mastitis, wound infection and deep vein thrombosis.

53. Answer **FTFFT**

Lichen sclerosus is a chronic inflammatory skin condition that is more commonly seen in women than in men. It is frequently seen in postmenopausal women. It is a condition usually affecting the genitals that may cause itching, pain, superficial dyspareunia and scarring. In women it may cause a white thickening of the vulval skin. Lichen sclerosus is associated with an increased risk of vulval intraepithelial neoplasia. A biopsy may be taken to confirm the diagnosis. Lichen sclerosus often responds to a strong topical steroid preparation.

54. Answer **FTTTF**

The following are risk factors for ectopic pregnancy: previous ectopic pregnancy, previous tubal surgery, pelvic inflammatory disease, adhesions caused by endometriosis and infertility treatment. If pregnancy should result from contraceptive failure with the progestogen-only pill or the intrauterine contraceptive device, the risk of ectopic pregnancy is greater than with other methods of contraception.

55. Answer **FFFTF**

The upper two-thirds of the cervix has columnar epithelium and the lower one-third has stratified squamous epithelium. An ectropion is caused when columnar epithelium extends around the external os. Cervical ectopy may be associated with puberty, pregnancy and the oral contraceptive pill. It is usually an asymptomatic condition but may present with bleeding. Nabothian cysts are often asymptomatic and are seen as multiple translucent or yellow lesions on the cervix. They usually represent areas of tissue re-growth.

56. Answer **TFFFF**

Acute appendicitis is the most common general surgical condition during pregnancy. The risk of appendicitis during pregnancy is equivalent to the risk in non-pregnant women of a similar age. Appendicitis may present with right lower quadrant pain, however, the gravid uterus may displace the appendix such that with increasing gestation pain may be felt in the right upper quadrant. Nausea, vomiting and fever may support the diagnosis. An infected appendix is more likely to perforate in the third trimester; this may be due to a delay in diagnosis. There is an increased risk of preterm labour especially if there is peritonitis.

57. Answer **FFTTT**

Heroin use during pregnancy increases the risk of intrauterine growth restriction, premature labour and stillbirth. Respiratory depression and symptoms of withdrawal may occur in the neonate. Methadone maintenance therapy provides stable dosing, reduces drug seeking behaviour and the risks associated with it.

58. Answer **TFFTT**

Advancing maternal age is associated with an increase in subfertility, stillbirth and miscarriage. There is also a greater risk of chromosomal abnormalities such as Down syndrome. Furthermore, hypertensive disorders and gestational diabetes occur more frequently in older mothers. Women over the age of 35 are more likely to have induced labour, epidural anaesthesia, instrumental delivery and Caesarean section.

59. Answer **TTFTT**

Women with inflammatory bowel disease (IBD) should ideally conceive whilst in remission and whilst taking folic acid supplementation according to the British Society of Gastroenterology (*IBD Section of the British Society of Gastroenterology*, 2004; Guidelines for the management of inflammatory bowel disease in adults, *Gut*, **53**(Suppl V):v1–v16). Generally, the risks from active disease outweigh the risks of the medication used to control IBD, therefore the British Society of Gastroenterology recommends that azathioprine and corticosteroids may be used during pregnancy. Pregnancy is an absolute contraindication for methotrexate use. Methotrexate is teratogenic and therefore contraception is needed during and for at least 3 months after methotrexate therapy in men and women. Women with severe IBD have an increased risk of preterm delivery.

60. Answer **FFFFF**

Antepartum haemorrhage (APH) is often defined as bleeding after the 24th week of pregnancy. It is more common in multiparous women than in primiparous women. APH may be due to placenta praevia, placental abruption, vasa praevia and uterine rupture. Placenta praevia may cause recurrent bleeding that is painless. Bleeding due to placental abruption is usually associated with abdominal pain and uterine contractions. Vaginal examination may cause significant bleeding in a mother with vasa praevia. After an episode of bleeding in a Rhesus-negative mother, prophylactic anti-D immunoglobulin should be given.

61. Answer **FFTFF**

The combined oral contraceptive pill may be started 3 weeks after birth if not breastfeeding; if it is started after this, additional precautions are necessary for the first 7 days. The progesterone-only pill may be started 3 weeks postpartum. In breastfeeding women it is recommended that the first dose of DMPA should be delayed until 6 weeks after birth. The subdermal implant Nexplanon may be given 3 weeks after delivery.

62. Answer **FTFTF**

Vertical transmission of hepatitis C occurs in <10% of cases. There is an increased risk of vertical transmission if viral load is high or there is co-infection with HIV. Antenatal hepatitis B screening is carried out in the UK. Screening for hepatitis C may be offered to intravenous drug users, women who are HIV-positive or have hepatitis B. Caesarean section does not reduce vertical transmission of hepatitis C, unless there is also HIV co-infection.

63. Answer **TFFFT**

Toxoplasmosis is caused by the protozoan *Toxoplasma gondii*. Transmission may occur through contact with domestic cat faeces and consumption of raw meat. Furthermore, vertical transmission may take place. There is a risk of vertical transmission if an acute infection is acquired during pregnancy; most fetal infections occur in the third trimester. Congenital toxoplasmosis is more severe if infection occurs in early pregnancy, features include chorioretinitis, intracranial calcification and hydrocephalus.

64. Answer **TFFTF**

- A first degree tear involves injury to the perineal/vaginal skin.
- A second degree tear involves injury to the perineum including the perineal muscles, with the anal sphincter remaining intact.
- A third degree tear refers to perineal injury with a partial or complete disruption of the anal sphincter muscles but without breach of the rectal mucosa.
- A fourth degree tear refers to perineal injury involving the anal sphincter muscles and breach of the rectal mucosa.

65. Answer **FTFFF**

Syphilis may be treated with benzathine benzylpenicillin, doxycycline or erythromycin. Uncomplicated gonorrhoea may be treated with cefixime (unlicensed) or ciprofloxacin. Ceftriaxone is used to treat pharyngeal gonorrhoea infection. Uncomplicated chlamydia may be treated with azithromycin as a single dose or a course of doxycycline or erythromycin. Pelvic inflammatory disease should be treated for at least 14 days with doxycycline, metronidazole and a single dose of intramuscular ceftriaxone. Ofloxacin and metronidazole is an alternate regimen for pelvic inflammatory disease.

66. Answer **FFFTF**

Gastroschisis is a congenital defect of the abdominal wall usually to the right side of the umbilical cord, it does not usually present with other congenital defects. There is no covering of abdominal contents with a membrane. Exomphalos is a congenital abnormality that may occur with other congenital defects. It is a condition where abdominal contents herniate into the umbilical cord; the abdominal contents are covered by a membrane. Both conditions may be visualised on ultrasonography and may be associated with raised maternal serum alpha-fetoprotein levels.

67. Answer **TFFFT**

Domestic violence in the family has an impact on children's emotional and psychological development; there may also be an increased risk of physical abuse. According to the Department of Health (2009; *Improving safety, reducing harm: Children, young people and domestic violence, A practical toolkit for front-line practitioners*), in up to one-third of cases domestic violence may start or escalate during pregnancy. Domestic violence in pregnancy may be associated with an increased risk of miscarriage. Domestic violence may continue after a violent relationship has ended. Alcohol misuse may be a contributory factor in domestic violence.

68. Answer **FFFTF**

Clomifene is an anti-oestrogen that may be used in the treatment of female infertility. Clomifene blocks oestrogen receptors in the hypothalamus which in turn causes gonadotrophin release. Clomifene therapy should be withdrawn if there is visual disturbance or ovarian hyperstimulation. Clomifene may cause hot flushes. It is given for a period of 5 days in one cycle; the Committee on Safety of Medicines (CSM) recommends that it should not be used for longer than six cycles.

69. Answer **FTFTT**

Patau syndrome is caused by trisomy 13. It is the most severe of the viable trisomies; most cases result in miscarriage or stillbirth. There is an increased risk of Patau syndrome with advancing maternal age. Holoprosencephaly, polydactyly, facial clefting and cardiac defects are features of Patau syndrome.

70. Answer **FTTFT**

Meconium aspiration may cause airways obstruction, chemical pneumonitis, in addition to surfactant dysfunction. It usually occurs as a result of fetal hypoxia. Passage of meconium rarely occurs below 34 weeks of gestation. There is an increased risk of passage of meconium in pre-eclampsia, oligohydramnios, cocaine use and cigarette smoking.

71. Answer **FFFTT**

The Apgar scar may be used to assess a baby at 1 and 5 minutes post-delivery. The maximum score is 10. It is a semi-objective measure that takes into account the colour of the baby, respiratory effort, muscle tone, heart rate and reflex irritability.

72. Answer **FFFTF**

There is an increased risk of venous thromboembolism associated with air travel during pregnancy. Therefore it is advisable to avoid dehydration. It is recommended that air travel is avoided in uncomplicated singleton pregnancies at the end of 36 weeks of gestation to avoid the risk of in-flight delivery. It is recommended that air travel is avoided in uncomplicated multiple pregnancies at 32 weeks of gestation according to the UK Civil Aviation Authority. At cabin altitude maternal haemoglobin is approximately 90% saturated. Fetal PaO_2 is maintained due to high fetal haematocrit and the increased oxygen-carrying potential of fetal haemoglobin.

73. Answer **TFFTF**

CA125 may be used as a marker in ovarian epithelial cancer and may be used to investigate women with a pelvic mass. It may be used to monitor patients for relapse in ovarian cancer. An elevated CA125 may be caused by intra-abdominal malignancies, endometriosis, pelvic inflammatory disease, pregnancy and ascites. CA125 is not used as a national screening test but has been used selectively in trials in high-risk women who have a family history of ovarian cancer.

74. Answer **FFFFT**

Sensitivity is the proportion of people with a disease that go on to be detected by a positive test (true positives). Specificity is the proportion of people who do not have a disease that then test negative for the condition (true negatives). A false negative is where the disease is present and the test is negative. A false positive is where the disease is absent and the test is positive.

75. Answer **FFFTT**

Automated readings tend to underestimate blood pressure during pregnancy, owing to cardiovascular changes. Therefore, automated measurements should be carried out only after calibration against a mercury sphygmomanometer. Korotkoff phase 5 is the appropriate measurement of diastolic blood pressure. During pregnancy, systolic blood pressure changes little, but diastolic pressure decreases by approximately 10 mmHg between 13 and 20 weeks of gestation. Pregnancy-induced hypertension refers to an elevated blood pressure without proteinuria presenting for the first time after 20 weeks of gestation. If there is persistent hypertension and proteinuria at 6 weeks postpartum, further investigation for renal disease is needed.

76. Answer **FFFFF**

Levonorgestrel and ulipristal are emergency hormonal contraceptives that should be taken as soon as possible after unprotected sexual intercourse. Levonorgestrel is licensed for use up to 72 hours; however, it may be used after this with reduced effectiveness. Ulipristal may be used within 120 hours of unprotected sexual intercourse. Ulipristal is as effective as levonorgestrel in preventing pregnancy, but it has not been compared with insertion of an intrauterine device. Another dose of ulipristal is recommended if a woman vomits within 3 hours of taking the first dose. Ulipristal is a prescription-only medication. Counselling includes explaining that barrier contraception should be used until the next period and that the next period may be early or late.

77. Answer **TFFFT**

Risks of abdominal hysterectomy include damage to the bladder and/or the ureter, blood loss requiring blood transfusion, wound infection, pain, urinary tract infection and ovarian failure. Bowel perforation, pelvic abscess formation and venous thromboembolism occur less commonly.

78. Answer **TTTFF**

According to the Fraser guidelines, a doctor may give contraceptive advice or treatment if the following criteria are fulfilled: a girl (<16 years) has capacity to make decisions, that the patient cannot be persuaded to inform her parents, that she is likely to have sexual intercourse with or without contraceptive treatment, that unless she is given advice/treatment her physical or mental health would be at risk, and giving treatment is in her best interests. Children under 13 years are not considered to have capacity to consent to sexual activity. If there are no concerns about the health, safety and welfare of a minor, confidentiality may be upheld.

79. Answer **TFFFF**

Bacterial vaginosis (BV) is caused by an overgrowth of anaerobic organisms as a result of an increase in pH in the vagina. It is more common in sexually active women but it is not considered a sexually transmitted infection. It is not usually associated with pain or itching, but an offensive fishy smelling vaginal discharge is characteristic. A thin, white or grey discharge may be seen. BV is associated with an increased risk of preterm birth.

80. Answer **TFFTF**

The vasomotor symptoms of the menopause may be triggered by alcohol, caffeine and spicy food. There is some evidence that selective serotonin re-uptake inhibitors may be used to treat menopausal symptoms but they are unlicensed for this use. Clonidine is licensed for the treatment of vasomotor symptoms of the menopause. There is no evidence that complementary therapies such as black cohosh, evening primrose oil and gingko biloba are effective.

81. Answer **FTFFF**

Medroxyprogesterone (Depo-Provera) is a long-acting progestogen. It is associated with an irregular bleeding pattern, delayed return of fertility and a reduction in bone mineral density. It is given by intramuscular injection within the first 5 days of a cycle every 12 weeks. If the interval is greater than 12 weeks and 5 days between injections, pregnancy should be excluded. Depo-Provera may be given within 5 days postpartum but there is an increased risk of heavy bleeding. In women who are breastfeeding, the injection should be delayed until 6 weeks postpartum.

82. Answer **FFTFF**

Pruritic urticated papules and plaques of pregnancy (PUPPP) usually appear in the 3rd trimester of a first pregnancy and the condition improves within a few days after delivery. An itchy rash usually appears initially on abdominal striae and then spreads to the limbs. Emollients, topical steroids and oral antihistamines may be used for symptomatic management. Direct immunofluorescence is negative. Pemphigoid gestationis is a rare blistering skin condition that occurs most commonly during the 2nd trimester but it may arise at any stage.

83. Answer **TFFFT**

Respiratory distress syndrome in the neonate is usually caused by the lack of alveolar surfactant in the lungs. There is an increased risk of respiratory distress syndrome with premature delivery, Caesarean section, maternal diabetes, multiple pregnancy, meconium aspiration and congenital diaphragmatic hernia. The risk may be reduced by administration of antenatal corticosteroids.

84. Answer **FFTFF**

Malaria during pregnancy is associated with an increased rate of miscarriage, premature birth and fetal growth restriction. A travel history should be sought in a pregnant woman presenting with pyrexia of unknown origin. The diagnosis is confirmed on thick and thin blood film examination or by detection of parasite antigen or enzyme. Maternal complications of malaria during pregnancy include anaemia, hypoglycaemia and acute pulmonary oedema (*RCOG*, 2010; *Green-top Guideline 54A: The prevention of malaria in pregnancy*).

85. Answer **FTFTT**

Natural family planning works on the basis of a woman predicting when she is likely to be fertile and abstaining from sexual intercourse during these times. Intercourse is avoided from 7 days before ovulation until 1–2 days after this as an ovum is likely to survive for 24 hours and a spermatozoan may survive for up to 7 days. Ovulation may be predicted by a slight increase in body temperature and a change in vaginal secretions. It may take up to six cycles to predict when to abstain from sexual intercourse. Natural family planning may be difficult if a woman has irregular periods.

86. Answer **FFFTF**

Vitamin K deficiency bleeding or haemorrhagic disease of the newborn results in a deficiency of clotting factors. Early vitamin K deficiency bleeding occurs within 24 hours of birth, and late vitamin K deficiency bleeding may occur between 2 and 12 weeks post-delivery. Babies that are breastfed are at increased risk of this condition when compared with formula-fed babies. Malabsorption of fat-soluble vitamins in conditions such as coeliac disease and cystic fibrosis may be contributory. It is recommended that all newborn babies receive vitamin K to prevent vitamin K deficiency bleeding; 1 mg may be given as a single intramuscular injection or two doses of phytomenadione may be given orally in the first week. A third dose is given as part of the oral regimen at 1 month for exclusively breastfed babies.

87. Answer **FFTFF**

Ovarian hyperstimulation syndrome (OHSS) is caused by induction of ovulation for the purpose of assisted conception. Mild OHSS affects up to 33% of *in vitro* fertilisation cycles. Symptoms may arise up to 5 days after egg harvesting. Severe OHSS may cause ascites, haemoconcentration and oliguria. There is an increased risk with younger women and those with polycystic ovary disease.

88. Answer **FFTFT**

Potter syndrome refers to a typical physical appearance of a neonate caused by oligohydramnios and compression whilst *in utero*. Characteristically there is a recessed chin, prominent epicanthal folds and low set ears. This may arise as a result of polycystic kidney disease, bilateral renal agenesis, posterior urethral valves and prolonged rupture of membranes. Oligohydramnios usually results in pulmonary hypoplasia which may cause respiratory distress at birth. Cardiac defects and musculoskeletal malformations such as clubbed feet and sacral agenesis may occur in association.

Exam paper 4

Extended matching questions

Options for questions 1–3

A	Colposcopy	F	5 year recall
B	Routine 3- or 5-yearly recall depending on age	G	Cytology at 6 months
C	Treatment	H	Sample tested for human papilloma virus (HPV)
D	3 year recall	I	For cytology at 1 year
E	Reassurance only	J	No treatment required

Instructions: for each of the scenarios given below, choose the **single** most appropriate option for the next management step from the list above. Each option may be used once, more than once or not at all.

Question 1	Low-grade dyskaryosis
Question 2	Low-grade dyskaryosis, HPV positive
Question 3	Low-grade dyskaryosis, negative colposcopy

Options for questions 4–6

A	Uterine artery Doppler	F	Testing for syphilis
B	Umbilical artery Doppler from 26–28 weeks of pregnancy	G	Serial measurement of symphysis fundal height
C	Umbilical artery Doppler from 30–34 weeks of pregnancy	H	Testing for parvovirus
D	Serial ultrasound with umbilical artery Doppler	I	Testing for malaria
E	Karyotyping and referral to a fetal medicine specialist	J	Referral to a fetal medicine specialist

Instructions: for each of the situations given below, choose the **single** most appropriate option for the next management step from the list above. Each option may be used once, more than once or not at all.

Question 4	Severe small-for-gestational-age fetus identified at anomaly scan, no structural abnormalities
Question 5	Severe small-for-gestational-age fetus identified at anomaly scan, structural abnormalities present
Question 6	Fetal echogenic bowel

Options for questions 7–9

A	5–10% of pregnancies	F	Nulliparity
B	Fetal growth restriction	G	Oligohydramnios
C	Diabetes	H	High body mass index (BMI)
D	Bleeding from or into the genital tract that occurs from 24 weeks of pregnancy	I	1–3% of pregnancies
E	Bleeding from or into the genital tract that occurs from 18–20 weeks of pregnancy	J	3–5% of pregnancies

Instructions: for each of the phrases given below, choose the **single** most appropriate answer from the list above. Each option may be used once, more than once or not at all.

Question 7	Definition of antepartum haemorrhage (APH)
Question 8	Percentage of pregnancies in which APH occurs as a complication
Question 9	A risk factor for placental abruption

Options for questions 10–12

A	hCG level	F	Reassurance
B	3-monthly ultrasound	G	Lactate dehydrogenase (LDH) level
C	Alpha-fetoprotein (AFP) level	H	CT scan
D	Midline laparotomy	I	6-monthly ultrasound
E	Laparoscopic surgery	J	Yearly ultrasound

Instructions: for each of the scenarios described below, choose the **single** most appropriate management option from the list above. Each option may be used once, more than once or not at all.

Question 10	Simple ovarian cysts 5–7 cm in diameter
Question 11	Simple ovarian cyst 8 cm in diameter that is symptomatic
Question 12	Simple ovarian cyst 2 cm in diameter

Options for questions 13–15

A	Reassurance	F	Screening for sexually transmitted infections
B	Amoxicillin	G	Endocervical swabs
C	Urgent screening for GBS	H	Clarithromycin
D	Caesarean section	I	Routine screening
E	Intrapartum antibiotic prophylaxis	J	Vaginal swabs

Instructions: for each of the scenarios described below, choose the **single** most appropriate option for the next management step from the list above. Each option may be used once, more than once or not at all.

Question 13	Vaginal colonisation with group B streptococcus (GBS) antenatally
Question 14	GBS bacteriuria
Question 15	Positive vaginal swab for GBS

Options for questions 16–18

A	CT scan	F	Epidural anaesthesia
B	Echocardiogram	G	Caesarean section
C	ECG	H	Assisted delivery
D	Chest X-ray	I	Five-fold
E	Three- to four-fold	J	Two-fold

Instructions: for each of the questions given below, choose the **single** most appropriate answer from the options above. Each option may be used once, more than once or not at all.

Question 16	Extent to which pregnancy increases the risk of acute myocardial infarction
Question 17	First-line investigation for all women with chest pain in pregnancy
Question 18	Investigation of choice in mitral valve stenosis

Options for questions 19–21

A	1%	F	After 11 weeks of gestation
B	2%	G	After 14 weeks of gestation
C	3%	H	Before 10 weeks of gestation
D	0.25%	I	0.5%
E	After 15 weeks of gestation	J	>1%

Instructions: for each of the scenarios given below, choose the **single** most appropriate option from the list above. Each option may be used once, more than once or not at all.

Question 19	The additional risk of miscarriage following amniocentesis
Question 20	The additional risk of miscarriage following chorionic villus sampling
Question 21	The timing of chorionic villus sampling

Options for questions 22–24

A	Weekly and ≥10 days postnatally	F	20%
B	Fortnightly and ≥1 month postnatally	G	1.5%
C	Every 72 hours	H	3%
D	In the postnatal period only	I	4%
E	50%	J	40%

Instructions: for each of the questions given below, choose the **single** most appropriate option from the list above. Each option may be used once, more than once or not at all.

Question 22	Percentage of women of Indian–Asian or Pakistani–Asian origin affected by obstetric cholestasis
Question 23	Percentage of pregnancies affected by pruritus
Question 24	Frequency of checking LFTs following diagnosis

Options for questions 25–27

A	16 weeks of gestation	F	Ultrasound scan assessment
B	20 weeks of gestation	G	28 weeks of gestation
C	Handheld Doppler device	H	30 weeks of gestation
D	CTG	I	32 weeks of gestation
E	Reassurance only	J	24 weeks of gestation

Instructions: for each of the situations given below, choose the **single** most appropriate option from the list above. Each option may be used once, more than once or not at all.

Question 25	When most women are aware of fetal movements
Question 26	When fetal movements may plateau
Question 27	Investigation of choice when, at 28 weeks of gestation, there have been reduced fetal movements, and a heartbeat can be auscultated

Options for questions 28–30

A	Intrauterine device	**F**	Mirena coil
B	Repeat hormone levels in 6 weeks	**G**	Check LH level
C	Continue progestogen-only contraception	**H**	Check FSH level
D	Consider HRT	**I**	No need for contraceptive cover
E	Switch to combined oral contraceptive pill	**J**	Continue condom use for at least 6 months

Instructions: for each of the patients described below, choose the **single** most appropriate management option from the list above. Each option may be used once, more than once or not at all.

Question 28	A 52 year old woman last had a period 6 months ago. She is reliably using condoms, and she does not wish to change her contraceptive method.
Question 29	A 49 year old woman last had a period 2 years ago; she is reliably using condoms.
Question 30	A 50 year old amenorrhoeic woman on Cerazette has an FSH level of 20.

Single best answer questions

31 Which one of the following statements about whooping cough is **true**?

  A Pertussis is caused by the Gram-positive organism *Bordetella pertussis*.

  B Protection conferred through vaccination is life-long.

  C Pregnant women are not at an increased risk of severe pertussis.

  D Pregnant women should be vaccinated in early pregnancy.

  E Vaccination against pertussis should not be combined with tetanus, diphtheria and polio.

32 Concerning Nexplanon, which one of the following options is **false**?

  A Nexplanon may be used for up to 3 years.

  B The implant contains etonogestrel which inhibits ovulation.

  C There is a rapid return to normal menstruation on implant removal.

  D Nexplanon should be inserted after the 4th week postpartum.

  E Amenorrhoea may occur in about 1 out of 3 women.

33 Regarding rubella, which one of the following statements is **false**?

  A Antenatal screening helps determine whether rubella may have occurred in the current pregnancy.

  B The infectious period is from 7 days before to 7 days after rash onset.

  C Rubella may be asymptomatic in up to 50% of cases.

  D The rash may be pruritic.

  E The risk to the fetus of primary rubella is significant, particularly in the first trimester.

34 Regarding diabetes, which one of the following statements is **false**?

A   Pregnancies affected by diabetes are associated with a higher risk of pre-eclampsia.

B   There is an increased risk of miscarriage in diabetic pregnancies.

C   Progestogens may increase insulin resistance.

D   Women who have had diabetes for less than 25 years, and have no end organ disease, may safely use all reversible methods of contraception.

E   Oestrogen should be avoided in diabetics with peripheral vascular disease.

35 Regarding subcutaneous depot medroxyprogesterone acetate, which one of the following statements is **false**?

A   It is bioequivalent to intramuscular depot medroxyprogesterone acetate.

B   This method of contraception prevents ovulation.

C   It may be associated with weight gain and a delayed return to fertility.

D   It is licensed for self-administration.

E   It is licensed to be administered at intervals of 13 weeks +/- 7 days.

36 Which one of the following is **not** a risk factor for postnatal depression?

A   Unemployment.

B   Previous psychiatric disorder.

C   Diet-controlled gestational diabetes.

D   Pre-eclampsia.

E   Emergency Caesarean section.

37 Which one of the following statements regarding miscarriage is **true**?

A Recurrent miscarriage is defined as the loss of two or more consecutive pregnancies.

B 20–30% of diagnosed pregnancies may result in early pregnancy loss.

C There is not an increased risk of miscarriage with advancing maternal age.

D Women with polycystic ovary syndrome have an increased risk of miscarriage.

E Uncontrolled diabetes is not a risk factor for recurrent miscarriage.

38 Which one of the following is **not** associated with second trimester miscarriages?

A Uterine septum.

B Depression.

C Bicornuate uterus.

D Bacterial vaginosis.

E Protein C deficiency.

39 Which one of the following statements is **true**?

A DVT during pregnancy often affects the right leg.

B D-dimer testing should be performed in pregnancy to diagnose acute venous thromboembolism.

C Duplex ultrasound is the first-line investigation if there is clinical suspicion of DVT.

D If there is a suspicion of PE, Doppler imaging should be considered first-line.

E The radiation dose to the fetus from computed tomography pulmonary angiogram (CTPA) is significant.

40 Regarding warfarin, which one of the following statements is **true**?

A   The risk of warfarin embryopathy may be minimised if the drug is avoided between 12 and 16 weeks of pregnancy.

B   The risk of warfarin embryopathy may be minimised if the drug is avoided between 16 and 20 weeks of pregnancy.

C   Warfarin during pregnancy may decrease the risk of nasal hypoplasia.

D   Warfarin during pregnancy does not increase the risk of miscarriage.

E   Warfarin during pregnancy may cause stippled epiphyses.

41 Regarding Zoely, which one of the following statements is **false**?

A   The mode of action is primarily on ovulation inhibition.

B   Nomegestrol acetate (NOMAC) has strong anti-gonadotrophic and mild anti-androgenic activity.

C   Zoely has fewer effects on lipid and glucose metabolism when compared to other combined oral contraceptives.

D   There is a 25/5 regimen with no pill-free interval.

E   There may be shorter and lighter withdrawal bleeding with Zoely.

42 Which one of the following statements is **true** regarding maternal request for Caesarean section (CS)?

A   All women who request CS should accept referral to a healthcare professional with expertise in providing perinatal mental health support.

B   If a woman declines perinatal mental health support a CS should not be offered.

C   An obstetrician unwilling to perform a CS should refer the woman to an obstetrician who will carry out the CS.

D Decision-to-delivery intervals are not helpful in measuring the overall performance of an obstetric unit.

E The decision-to-delivery interval for a category 1 CS should be 40 minutes.

43 Which one of the following statements is **true**?

A Prophylactic antibiotics should be given before skin incision at Caesarean section.

B Prophylactic antibiotics should be given after skin incision at Caesarean section.

C Endometritis, urinary tract and wound infection may occur in approximately 15% of women who have had a CS.

D Endometritis, urinary tract and wound infection may occur in approximately 25% of women who have had a CS.

E The risk of fever, bladder injuries and surgical injuries does not vary with planned mode of birth in women who have had ≥3 Caesarean sections.

44 Which one of the following statements regarding chronic pelvic pain is **false**?

A Pelvic pain which is variable over the menstrual cycle may be hormonally driven.

B Eliciting a history of dysmenorrhoea and dyspareunia may be helpful.

C Bladder and bowel symptoms should be considered.

D Sexually active women with chronic pelvic pain should be offered screening for sexually transmitted infections.

E There is good evidence to support division of adhesions in women with chronic pelvic pain.

45 Regarding shoulder dystocia, which one of the following statements is **incorrect**?

A Shoulder dystocia is associated with a prolonged first stage of labour.

B Shoulder dystocia is associated with a prolonged second stage of labour.

C There is an increased risk of shoulder dystocia with maternal body mass index <28.

D There is an increased risk of shoulder dystocia with oxytocin augmentation.

E There is an increased risk of shoulder dystocia with assisted vaginal delivery.

46 Regarding bacterial sepsis following pregnancy, which one of the following statements is **true**?

A The most common site of sepsis in the puerperium is the urinary tract.

B Hypothermia is not a sign of sepsis.

C Cervical cerclage is not a risk factor for sepsis in the puerperium.

D Oliguria is not a sign of sepsis.

E Being black or of minority ethnic group origin increases the risk of bacterial sepsis in the puerperium.

47 Which one of the following statements is **false**?

A Small-for-gestational-age (SGA) refers to an infant born with a birth weight less than the 10th centile.

B SGA refers to an infant born with a birth weight less than the 15th centile.

C Up to 70% of SGA fetuses may be constitutionally small.

D Women who have a major risk factor for SGA should be referred for serial ultrasound with umbilical artery Doppler from 26–28 weeks.

E Women who have three or more minor risk factors should be referred for uterine artery Doppler at 20–24 weeks of gestation.

48 Which one of the following statements is **true**?

A   Previous Caesarean section is not a risk factor for placenta praevia.

B   Multiple pregnancy decreases the risk of placenta praevia.

C   Smoking does not increase the risk of placenta praevia.

D   Multiparity increases the risk of placenta praevia.

E   Termination of pregnancy does not increase the risk of placenta praevia.

Multiple choice questions

For each of these multiple choice questions, you must indicate which of the statements are true and which are false.

49 Concerning cervical screening

A If there are borderline changes or low-grade dyskaryosis, the sample is not tested for human papilloma virus (HPV).

B If there are borderline changes and the sample is HPV-positive, the patient is invited for colposcopy.

C If treatment is required for CIN 1, cytology is repeated at 12 months.

D For CIN 2/3, cytology is repeated at 6 months after treatment.

E Following borderline changes and negative colposcopy, routine 5-year recall is initiated.

50 Concerning severe small-for-gestational-age

A If severe SGA is identified at the 18–20 week scan, a referral to a fetal medicine specialist should be offered.

B Karyotyping should be offered in severely SGA fetuses, particularly if structural anomalies are present.

C Serological screening for congenital cytomegalovirus (CMV) should not be offered.

D Toxoplasmosis screening should be considered.

E Testing for syphilis and malaria should be routinely considered.

51 Placental abruption may be associated with the following:

A Pre-eclampsia.

B Polyhydramnios.

C Low body mass index (BMI).

D Domestic violence.

E Cocaine use during pregnancy.

52 Concerning ovarian cysts

A Simple ovarian cysts which are <5 cm diameter usually resolve over 2–3 menstrual cycles.

B Women with simple ovarian cysts of 7–10 cm in diameter should have yearly ultrasound follow-up.

C Serum Ca-125 needs to be undertaken in all premenopausal women with simple ovarian cysts.

D Lactate dehydrogenase (LDH) and hCG should be measured in all women under age 40 with a complex ovarian mass.

E AFP should be measured in all women under age 40 with a complex ovarian mass.

53 Group B streptococcus (GBS)

A GBS is screened for routinely.

B Antenatal prophylaxis with oral benzylpenicillin for vaginal / rectal colonisation reduces the risk of GBS colonisation at delivery.

C Intrapartum antibiotic prophylaxis does not need to be offered to women with GBS bacteriuria.

D Intrapartum antibiotic prophylaxis should be offered to women who are pyrexial in labour.

E Benzylpenicillin should be administered after the onset of labour and given regularly until delivery.

54 Concerning subcutaneous depot medroxyprogesterone acetate

A It is bioequivalent to intramuscular depot medroxyprogesterone acetate.

B It prevents fertilisation.

C It may be associated with amenorrhoea.

D There may be a delayed return to fertility.

E It may be self-administered.

55 Concerning Zoely

A Its mode of action is primarily on ovulation inhibition.

B It has more adverse effects on lipid and glucose metabolism when compared to other combined oral contraceptives.

C There is a 25/5 regimen with no pill-free interval.

D 5 days of active (white) tablets are needed to maintain ovulation suppression.

E Zoely may be taken continuously to delay withdrawal bleeding.

56 Concerning amniocentesis and chorionic villus sampling (CVS)

A The additional risk of miscarriage following amniocentesis is approximately 2%.

B Amniocentesis should be performed after 15 weeks of gestation.

C Early amniocentesis has an increased risk of fetal talipes.

D CVS should not be performed before 12 completed weeks of gestation.

E CVS is usually performed between 11 and 13 weeks of gestation.

57 Concerning vulval skin disorders

A Women with lichen sclerosus are at increased risk of autoimmune disorders.

B Women with erosive lichen planus are at increased risk of autoimmune disorders.

C Skin biopsy is necessary.

D Skin biopsy is required if the woman fails to respond to treatment.

E Women with vulval skin disorders require examination of other mucosal sites.

58 Antenatal corticosteroids

A Women between 24 and 34^{+6} weeks of gestation who are at risk of preterm birth should be offered antenatal corticosteroids routinely.

B Women between 23 and 23^{+6} weeks of gestation who are at risk of preterm birth should be offered antenatal corticosteroids routinely.

C Women with multiple pregnancy between 24 and 34^{+6} weeks of gestation who are at risk of preterm birth should be offered antenatal corticosteroids routinely.

D If Caesarean section is planned at 38^{+6} weeks of gestation, antenatal corticosteroids should be offered.

E If Caesarean section is planned at 39 weeks of gestation, antenatal corticosteroids should be offered.

59 Outpatient hysteroscopy

A Women should be advised to consider taking opiates approximately 1 hour before their outpatient hysteroscopy to reduce post-operative pain.

B Topical local anaesthesia should be considered if a cervical tenaculum is to be used.

C Local anaesthesia in the cervical canal helps to reduce pain.

D Local anaesthesia in the cervical canal may reduce the incidence of vasovagal reactions.

E Conscious sedation may be used routinely.

60 Concerning smoking during pregnancy

A Smoking during pregnancy does not affect the risk of premature delivery.

B Smoking does not increase the risk of stillbirth.

C Smoking increases the risk of sudden infant death syndrome.

D Infants of parents who smoke are more likely to suffer from asthma.

E Infants of parents who smoke are less likely to suffer from glue ear.

61 Amniotic fluid embolism:

A May occur following termination of pregnancy.

B May occur following placental abruption.

C May be associated with advanced maternal age.

D May be associated with multiparity.

E May present with acute shortness of breath and hypotension.

62 Regarding echogenic bowel

A Echogenic bowel is seen in 2% of pregnancies.

B It may be associated with cytomegalovirus infection.

C It is not associated with intrauterine growth restriction.

D It is not associated with chromosome anomalies.

E Most fetuses identified with echogenic bowel are normal.

63 Regarding club-foot

A Club-foot may be syndromic.

B It may be associated with polyhydramnios.

C It may be associated with uterine anomalies.

D Female fetuses are predominantly affected.

E The highest rates are seen in Asian populations.

64 Phenylketonuria (PKU):

A Is an X-linked recessive disorder.

B Is part of the newborn blood spot programme.

C May be caused by an enzyme deficiency.

D Is caused by low levels of phenylalanine.

E Presents shortly after birth.

65 Regarding urinary tract infections in pregnancy

A   Pregnant women are at increased risk for UTIs, particularly in the 1st trimester.

B   An increased risk may be attributable to ureteral dilatation and decreased ureteral tone.

C   There is an increased risk due to increased bladder tone.

D   Up to 20% of pregnant women develop glycosuria.

E   Glycosuria increases the risk of UTIs in pregnancy.

66 Cardiovascular changes in pregnancy

A   Cardiac output is increased by up to 30%.

B   Stroke volume does not increase.

C   Peripheral vascular resistance decreases.

D   Heart rate remains unchanged whilst contractility of the heart increases.

E   The cardiac apex is displaced to the right.

67 Aortocaval compression

A   In the supine position the gravid uterus may reduce cardiac output.

B   Uteroplacental blood flow is reduced in the supine position.

C   Renal blood flow is unaffected in the supine position.

D   Right lateral tilt is required for Caesarean section.

E   Epidural blocks may worsen supine hypotension.

68 Concerning the menstrual cycle

A   The hypothalamus secretes gonadotrophin-releasing hormone (GnRH), which stimulates the posterior pituitary gland.

B   Follicle-stimulating hormone (FSH) causes an ovarian dominant follicle to grow.

C   Mid-cycle there is a surge of luteinising hormone (LH).

D Mid-cycle there is a surge of FSH.

E FSH and LH levels decrease when the ovum is released.

69 Tranexamic acid:

A Is a non-competitive inhibitor of the activation of plasminogen to plasmin.

B May be used to treat dysmenorrhoea.

C May be started prior to menstruation.

D Is not contraindicated if there is a history of venous thrombosis.

E Is contraindicated if there is a history of arterial thrombosis.

70 Concerning ovarian cancer, the following are risk factors:

A Multiparity.

B Family history.

C BRCA1 gene mutation.

D BRCA2 gene mutation.

E Hereditary non-polyposis colorectal cancer.

71 Regarding BRCA1 and 2 gene mutations

A BRCA1 and 2 gene mutations are associated with an increased risk of breast cancer.

B There is a 10% risk of ovarian cancer if a close relative is affected.

C Women with BRCA2 gene mutation have a 40–60% lifetime risk of developing ovarian cancer.

D Women with BRCA1 gene mutation have a 10–30% lifetime risk of developing ovarian cancer.

E The risk of developing ovarian cancer starts to increase from the age of 40 for BRCA1 carriers and in the mid 40s for BRCA2 carriers.

72 Parvovirus B19 and pregnancy

A Parvovirus B19 usually causes a severe illness in a pregnant woman.

B Parvovirus B19 infection in the first 20 weeks of pregnancy may cause intrauterine death.

C Parvovirus B19 infection in the first 20 weeks of pregnancy may cause fetal anaemia.

D Up to two-thirds of women are seronegative for parvovirus B19.

E There is a screening programme for parvovirus B19.

73 Symptoms suggestive of ovarian cancer include:

A Bloating.

B Pelvic pain.

C Urinary urgency.

D Urinary frequency.

E Abdominal pain.

74 Blood vessels

A The uterine artery arises directly from the abdominal aorta.

B The uterine artery arises from the internal iliac artery.

C The right ovarian vein terminates in the inferior vena cava.

D The left ovarian vein usually terminates in the inferior vena cava.

E The ovarian fossa is located between the external and internal iliac vessels.

75 Pelvic lymphatics

A Most of the lymph from the pelvis drains into nodes adjacent to the external iliac artery.

B Lymph nodes adjacent to the internal iliac artery drain into the common iliac nodes.

C Lymphatic vessels from the ovaries drain into nodes adjacent to the internal iliac artery.

D Lymphatic vessels from the rectum pass directly to the aortic nodes.

E Some vessels from the body of the uterus drain into the superficial inguinal nodes.

76 Pharmacotherapy for smoking cessation in pregnancy and whilst breastfeeding

A Women should ideally stop smoking without using nicotine replacement therapy.

B Nicotine exposure in breast milk is significant.

C Pregnant and breastfeeding women who are using nicotine patches to aid smoking cessation should be advised to change them before going to bed.

D Bupropion is recommended for use in women who are pregnant or breastfeeding.

E Varenicline is recommended for use in women who are pregnant or breastfeeding.

77 Vulval skin conditions

A Up to 10% of women with anogenital lichen sclerosus will have steroid-resistant disease.

B Up to 20% of women with anogenital lichen sclerosus will have steroid-resistant disease.

C Steroid-resistant disease may be managed with topical tacrolimus in general practice.

D Women who have been treated for VIN are at risk of intraepithelial neoplasia at other sites.

E The gold standard for the treatment of VIN is local surgical excision.

78 Zoladex:

A Is used in the management of endometriosis.

B May be used prior to endometrial ablation.

C May be used prior to endometrial resection.

D May be used prior to fibroid surgery.

E May cause loss of bone mineral density.

79 Vaginismus:

A Refers to recurrent or persistent involuntary spasm of the musculature of the outer third of the vagina which may interfere with intercourse.

B Does not affect the ability to use tampons.

C May be caused by vestibulitis.

D May be related to sexual assault.

E May be treated by using graded vaginal trainers.

80 Depo-Provera and bone mineral density

A It is not recommended that, for women with significant lifestyle and/or medical risk factors for osteoporosis, other methods of contraception should be considered.

B Depo-Provera is associated with a small loss of bone mineral density, which is not usually recovered after discontinuation.

C There is no available evidence on the effect on long-term fracture risk.

D Depo-Provera use should be re-evaluated on a yearly basis.

E Re-evaluation includes bone density measurement in menopausal women.

81 The ovary

A The ovaries are suspended with the posterior surfaces of the broad ligaments.

B Most of the ovarian surface is covered in peritoneum.

C The ovary lies in the ovarian fossa, between the external and internal iliac vessels.

D The ureter descends in the posterior boundary of the ovarian fossa.

E The ovarian artery arises from the internal iliac artery.

82 Hereditary non-polyposis colorectal cancer (HNPCC):

A Is an autosomal recessive condition.

B Is caused by a germline mutation in one of several DNA mismatch repair genes.

C May cause up to 10% of colorectal malignancies.

D May cause up to 5% of endometrial cancers.

E Women with HNPCC may have an up to 70% risk of endometrial cancer.

83 Risk factors for endometrial cancer include:

A Multiparity.

B Early menopause.

C Family history of endometrial cancer.

D Polycystic ovarian disease.

E Hereditary non-polyposis colorectal cancer (HNPCC).

84 Renal physiology during pregnancy

A Glomerular filtration rate increases.

B Renal plasma flow is unchanged.

C Plasma urea and creatinine is lower in pregnancy.

D Plasma osmolality is unchanged.

E Proteinuria can occur in normal pregnancy.

85 The circulation during pregnancy

A Blood volume continues to increase until 37 weeks.

B Plasma volume increases by 30%.

C Red cell mass increases by 20–30%.

D Total body water increases.

E The white cell count and platelet count increase during pregnancy.

86 Obstetric cholestasis

A Pruritus in obstetric cholestasis usually involves the palms and soles of the feet.

B Pruritus in obstetric cholestasis is usually worse during the day.

C There is an increased risk of meconium passage associated with obstetric cholestasis.

D There is an increased risk of stillbirth.

E There is an increased risk of premature birth.

87 Antenatal corticosteroids:

A Reduce neonatal death rates.

B Reduce the risk of respiratory distress syndrome.

C Reduce the risk of intraventricular haemorrhage.

D Have no known benefits for the mother.

E Should be given to women for whom an elective Caesarean section is planned prior to 39 weeks of gestation.

88 Vulval dermatitis

A Women presenting with vulval dermatitis should be assessed for symptoms of urinary incontinence.

B Women presenting with vulval dermatitis do not need to be assessed for symptoms of faecal incontinence.

C The history should include details of any personal or family history of atopic conditions.

D It is not helpful to check serum ferritin.

E Skin patch testing should be performed for women seen with vulval dermatitis.

Answers and explanations for exam paper 4

1. Answer **H** Sample tested for human papilloma virus (HPV)

2. Answer **A** Colposcopy

3. Answer **B** Routine 3- or 5-yearly recall depending on age

HPV triage and test of cure has been introduced in the cervical screening programme in England. If there are borderline changes or low-grade dyskaryosis, the sample is tested for human papilloma virus (HPV). If the sample is HPV-positive, the patient is invited for colposcopy. In the case of CIN 1, if no treatment is required cytology is repeated at 12 months. If treatment is required for CIN 1, cytology is repeated at 6 months. For CIN 2/3, cytology is repeated at 6 months after treatment. Following borderline changes and negative colposcopy, routine 3- or 5-year recall is resumed (*HPV triage and test of cure*, available at www.cancerscreening.nhs.uk/cervical/hpv-triage-test-of-cure.html [last accessed 5 September 2013]).

4. Answer **J** Referral to a fetal medicine specialist

5. Answer **E** Karyotyping and referral to a fetal medicine specialist

6. Answer **D** Serial ultrasound with umbilical artery Doppler

Small-for-gestational-age (SGA) is defined as an estimated fetal weight or abdominal circumference less than the 10th centile. If severe SGA is identified at the 18–20 week scan, a referral to a fetal medicine specialist should be offered. Karyotyping should be offered in severely SGA fetuses, particularly if structural anomalies are present. Serological screening for congenital cytomegalovirus (CMV) and toxoplasmosis infection should also be offered in severe SGA. Testing for syphilis and malaria should be considered in high risk populations.

Serial measurement of symphysis fundal height is recommended at each antenatal appointment from 24 weeks of pregnancy. Women who have a major risk factor should be referred for serial ultrasound with umbilical artery Doppler from 26–28 weeks of pregnancy.

Women who have three or more minor risk factors should be referred for uterine artery Doppler at 20–24 weeks of gestation. Minor risk factors include:

maternal age >40, nulliparity, smoking, daily vigorous exercise, previous stillbirth and previous pre-eclampsia. Serial ultrasound measurement of fetal size and assessment of wellbeing with umbilical artery Doppler should be offered in cases of fetal echogenic bowel (*RCOG*, 2013; Green-top Guideline 31: *The investigation and management of the small-for-gestational-age fetus*).

7. Answer D Bleeding from or into the genital tract that occurs from 24 weeks of pregnancy

8. Answer J 3–5% of pregnancies

9. Answer B Fetal growth restriction

Antepartum haemorrhage (APH) is defined as bleeding from or into the genital tract that occurs from 24 weeks of pregnancy. APH complicates 3–5% of pregnancies. Placenta praevia, placental abruption and local causes where there may be bleeding from the vulva, vagina or cervix may cause APH.

Risk factors for placental abruption include: pre-eclampsia, fetal growth restriction, polyhydramnios, advanced maternal age, multiparity, low body mass index (BMI), pregnancy following assisted reproductive techniques, intrauterine infection, premature rupture of membranes, abdominal trauma and smoking as well as cocaine and amphetamine use during pregnancy (*RCOG*, 2011; Green-top Guideline 63: *Antepartum haemorrhage*).

10. Answer J Yearly ultrasound

11. Answer E Laparoscopic surgery

12. Answer F Reassurance

Functional or simple ovarian cysts which are <5 cm diameter usually resolve over 2–3 menstrual cycles. Women with simple ovarian cysts of 5–7 cm in diameter should have yearly ultrasound follow-up and those with larger simple cysts should be considered for either further imaging (MRI) or surgical intervention. A laparoscopic approach is favoured for the management of benign ovarian masses. Symptoms that may suggest ovarian malignancy include: persistent abdominal distension, increased satiety, pelvic or abdominal pain. A serum Ca-125 does not need to be undertaken in all premenopausal women when a simple ovarian cyst has been diagnosed on ultrasound. Lactate dehydrogenase (LDH), AFP and hCG should be measured in all women under age 40 with a complex ovarian mass due to the risk of germ cell tumours (*RCOG/BSGE*, 2011; Joint Guideline 62: *Management of suspected ovarian masses in premenopausal women*).

13. Answer **A** Reassurance

14. Answer **E** Intrapartum antibiotic prophylaxis

15. Answer **E** Intrapartum antibiotic prophylaxis

Routine screening of all pregnant women for antenatal group B streptococcus (GBS) carriage is not recommended. Antenatal prophylaxis with oral benzylpenicillin for vaginal / rectal colonisation does not reduce the risk of GBS colonisation at delivery. Intrapartum antibiotic prophylaxis should be offered to women with GBS bacteriuria. Vaginal swabs should not be taken during pregnancy unless there is a clinical indication to do so. If these are positive for GBS, intrapartum antibiotic prophylaxis should be offered. Antibiotic prophylaxis specifically for GBS is not required for women undergoing planned Caesarean section in the absence of labour and with intact membranes. Intrapartum antibiotic prophylaxis should be offered to women who are pyrexial in labour (>38°C). For women who have accepted antibiotic therapy, benzylpenicillin should be administered after the onset of labour and given regularly until delivery. Clindamycin may be used in those who are penicillin-allergic (*RCOG*, 2012; Green-top Guideline 36: *The prevention of early-onset neonatal group B streptococcal disease*).

16. Answer **E** Three- to four-fold

17. Answer **C** ECG

18. Answer **B** Echocardiogram

Pregnancy may increase the risk of acute myocardial infarction three- to four-fold. All women with chest pain in pregnancy should have an ECG performed. Peripartum cardiomyopathy may present late in pregnancy or in the puerperium. Peripartum cardiomyopathy should be considered in any pregnant or puerperal woman who reports increasing shortness of breath, especially on lying flat or at night. These women should have an ECG, a chest X-ray and an echocardiogram performed. Rheumatic heart disease should be considered particularly in those women not born in the UK, mitral valve stenosis is the most common lesion. Early incremental epidural anaesthesia and assisted vaginal delivery may minimise cardiovascular stress. Caesarean section is usually only necessary for obstetric indications (*RCOG*, 2011; Good Practice 13: *Cardiac disease and pregnancy*).

19. Answer **A** 1%

20. Answer **J** >1%

21. Answer **F** After 11 weeks of gestation

The additional risk of miscarriage following amniocentesis is approximately 1%. Women should be advised that the additional risk of miscarriage following chorionic villus sampling (CVS) may be slightly higher than that of amniocentesis carried out after 15 weeks of gestation. CVS should not be performed before 10 completed weeks of gestation. CVS is usually performed between 11 and 13 weeks of gestation.

22. Answer **G** 1.5%

23. Answer **F** 20%

24. Answer **A** Weekly and ≥10 days postnatally

In England, obstetric cholestasis affects up to 1.5% of women of Indian–Asian or Pakistani–Asian origin. Obstetric cholestasis is diagnosed when unexplained pruritus occurs in pregnancy and there are abnormal liver function tests (LFTs) and/or raised bile acids. Pruritus in obstetric cholestasis usually involves the palms and soles of the feet, and it is usually worse at night. Pruritus in pregnancy may affect up to 23% of pregnancies. Following diagnosis, LFTs may be checked weekly and after at least 10 days postnatally. Postnatal resolution of pruritus and abnormal LFTs should be confirmed (*RCOG*, 2001; Green-top Guideline 43: *Obstetric cholestasis*).

25. Answer **B** 20 weeks of gestation

26. Answer **I** 32 weeks of gestation

27. Answer **D** CTG

Most women are aware of fetal movements by 20 weeks of gestation. Fetal movements may plateau at 32 weeks of gestation; however, there is no reduction in the frequency of fetal movements in the late third trimester. If a woman presents with reduced fetal movements, the fetal heart should be auscultated using a handheld Doppler device to exclude fetal death. If there is a heartbeat and there has been a decrease in fetal movements, a CTG should be performed to exclude fetal compromise if the pregnancy is over 28 weeks of gestation. If CTG is normal or there are additional risk factors for growth restriction / stillbirth and there is still concern about reduced fetal movements, an ultrasound scan assessment should be done (*RCOG*, 2011; Green-top Guideline 57: *Reduced fetal movements*).

28. Answer **J** Continue condom use for at least 6 months

29. Answer I No need for contraceptive cover

30. Answer C Continue progestogen-only contraception

Women who are not using hormonal contraception and who continue to have regular menses at the age of 55 years should continue with some form of contraception. Non-hormonal contraception can be stopped 1 year after the last menstrual period in those aged over 50 years, and 2 years after the last menstrual period in those under 50. Women over the age of 50 years who are amenorrhoeic and wish to stop progestogen-only contraception can have their FSH levels checked. If the level is ≥30 IU/L the FSH should be repeated after 6 weeks. If the second FSH level is ≥30 IU/L contraception can be stopped after 1 year. It is recommended that the combined oral contraceptive pill can be continued up to age 50 years and then switched to a non-hormonal or progestogen-only method.

31. Answer C

Pertussis is a respiratory infection characterised by a paroxysmal cough caused by the Gram-negative organism *Bordetella pertussis*. The current immunisation schedule is thought to provide protection in children until at least 10 years of age. The risk for pregnant women is in late pregnancy and relates to the potential of transmission to the newborn. Pregnant women in themselves do not appear to be at increased risk of severe pertussis. The Joint Committee on Vaccination and Immunisation (JCVI) has recommended a temporary programme of immunisation of women in the later stages of pregnancy. The rationale of this is to boost antibodies in vaccinated women in late pregnancy which will result in pertussis-specific antibodies being passed from mother to baby. Vaccination against pertussis, combined with tetanus, diphtheria and polio (Repevax) should be provided for all pregnant women, ideally between 28 and 38 weeks of pregnancy (*Pertussis Guideline Working Group*, 2012: *HPA guidelines for the public health management of pertussis incidents in healthcare settings*).

32. Answer E

Nexplanon is a subdermal implant that is a LARC which may be used for up to 3 years. It is a radio-opaque, progestogen-only implant. The implant contains etonogestrel which inhibits ovulation; in addition it causes changes in cervical mucus. The contraceptive action of etonogestrel is reversible and on removal of the implant there is a rapid return to normal menstruation. Nexplanon may be used during lactation and should be inserted after the 4th postpartum week. The major disadvantage of this method of contraception is that women are likely to have changes in their menstrual bleeding pattern. Amenorrhoea may occur in about one-fifth of women while another one-fifth may experience frequent and/or prolonged bleeding.

33. Answer E

There is routine antenatal testing for rubella antibody (IgG) as well as an immunisation schedule in the form of the measles, mumps and rubella (MMR) vaccine. Antenatal screening does not determine whether rubella may have occurred in the current pregnancy. The infectious period is from 7 days before to 7 days after rash onset. Rubella may be asymptomatic in up to 50% of cases but may present with prodromal symptoms such as low-grade pyrexia, conjunctivitis, sore throat, malaise and tender lymphadenopathy. The prodrome may last 1 to 5 days before the onset of a scarletiniform rash, which may be mildly pruritic. The risk to the fetus of primary rubella is significant, particularly in the first trimester. Fetal rubella syndrome includes intrauterine growth restriction, intracranial calcification, deafness, cataracts and cardiac defects (*HPA Rash Guidance Working Group*, 2011: *Guidance on viral rash in pregnancy: investigation, diagnosis and management of viral rash illness, or exposure to viral rash illness in pregnancy*).

34. Answer D

Pregnancies affected by diabetes result in a higher risk of miscarriage, congenital anomalies, pre-eclampsia and macrosomia. Women who have had diabetes for less than 20 years, and have no end organ disease, may safely use all reversible methods of contraception, according to both the World Health Organization and the US Centers for Disease Control and Prevention (CDC). Progestogens may increase insulin resistance but this is not thought to be clinically significant. Contraceptive options are more limited in diabetics who have vascular complications such as retinopathy, nephropathy, peripheral vascular disease and heart disease; in these cases oestrogen should be avoided.

35. Answer D

Subcutaneous depot medroxyprogesterone acetate is a progestogen-only injectable contraceptive, licensed for subcutaneous use, which is bioequivalent to intramuscular depot medroxyprogesterone acetate (150 mg Depo-Provera). It has recently been released in the UK. This method of contraception prevents ovulation. Both these methods may be associated with loss of bone mineral density, amenorrhoea, weight gain and a delayed return to fertility. It is licensed to be administered at intervals of 13 weeks +/- 7days. Advantages of subcutaneous administration include the potential for self-administration and a reduction in the likelihood of haematomas in patients with bleeding disorders or on anticoagulation. Self-administration is outside product licence (*Faculty of Sexual & Reproductive Healthcare*, 2013: *New product review from the clinical effectiveness unit: subcutaneous depot medroxyprogesterone acetate (Sayana Press)*).

36. Answer C

Postnatal depression may be associated with a previous psychiatric disorder, lack of supportive relationships, recent life events such as bereavement, unemployment and unplanned pregnancy. Other risk factors for developing postnatal depression include pre-eclampsia, hospitalisation during pregnancy, emergency Caesarean section and admission of the baby to special care (*NICE*, 2007; *Antenatal and postnatal mental health: Clinical management and service guidance*: CG45).

37. Answer D

Recurrent miscarriage is defined as the loss of three or more consecutive pregnancies. Spontaneous miscarriages may occur in up to half of pregnancies before the first missed menstrual period; 10–20% of diagnosed pregnancies may result in early pregnancy loss. There is an increased risk of miscarriage with advancing maternal age. Uncontrolled diabetes mellitus, systemic lupus erythematosus and thyroid disease may be risk factors for recurrent miscarriage. Women with polycystic ovary syndrome have an increased risk of miscarriage.

38. Answer B

Second-trimester miscarriages may be linked to uterine malformations such as presence of uterine septum or bicornuate uterus. All women with recurrent first-trimester miscarriage and all women with one or more second-trimester miscarriages should have a pelvic ultrasound to assess uterine anatomy. Bacterial vaginosis in the first trimester of pregnancy is a risk factor for second-trimester miscarriage and preterm delivery. Women with second-trimester miscarriage should be screened for inherited thrombophilias.

39. Answer C

DVT during pregnancy often affects the left leg due to left common iliac vein compression which is exacerbated by pressure from the gravid uterus. D-dimer testing should not be performed in pregnancy to diagnose acute venous thromboembolism. Duplex ultrasound is the first-line investigation if there is clinical suspicion of DVT. If there is a suspicion of PE, the RCOG recommend a chest X-ray in the first instance followed by compression duplex Doppler if the chest X-ray is normal. If both these tests are negative, a ventilation-perfusion (V/Q) scan or a computed tomography pulmonary angiogram (CTPA) should be considered. Chest X-ray and V/Q scanning are associated with negligible radiation to the fetus. The radiation dose to the fetus from CTPA is minimal but there is significant radiation to the maternal breasts.

40. Answer **E**

Women who are on warfarin should ideally have pre-pregnancy counselling about the risk of warfarin embryopathy so that they may be changed to low-molecular-weight heparin (LMWH) if appropriate. The risk of warfarin embryopathy may be minimised if the drug is avoided between 6 and 12 weeks of pregnancy. Warfarin crosses the placenta and causes an increased risk of congenital abnormalities such as nasal hypoplasia and/or stippled epiphyses, miscarriage, fetal haemorrhage and stillbirth.

41. Answer **D**

The new combined oral contraceptive pill Zoely became available in the UK in May 2013. Its mode of action is primarily on ovulation inhibition by suppression of gonadotrophins, as is the case with other combined hormonal contraceptives. It contains 1.5 mg 17β-estradiol and 2.5 mg nomegestrol acetate (NOMAC) per active tablet. NOMAC is a progestogen with strong anti-gonadotrophic and mild anti-androgenic activity. Current evidence suggests that Zoely has fewer effects on lipid and glucose metabolism when compared to other combined oral contraceptives. A white active tablet is taken for 24 days and an inactive yellow one for 4 days, that is, there is a 24/4 regimen with no pill-free interval. This results in shorter and lighter withdrawal bleeding; indeed withdrawal bleeds may be absent (*Faculty of Sexual & Reproductive Healthcare*, 2013; *Faculty statement from the clinical effectiveness unit: estradiol / nomegestrol combined pill, Zoely*).

42. Answer **C**

When a woman requests a CS due to anxiety about childbirth, a referral to a healthcare professional with expertise in providing perinatal mental health support should be offered. A planned CS may be offered if a vaginal birth would not be an acceptable option after a discussion and an offer of further support. An obstetrician unwilling to perform a CS should refer the woman to an obstetrician who will carry out the CS. Decision-to-delivery intervals may be helpful in measuring the overall performance of an obstetric unit. This should be 30 minutes for category 1 CS (*NICE*, 2011).

43. Answer **A**

Prophylactic antibiotics should be given before skin incision at Caesarean section. Endometritis, urinary tract and wound infection may occur in approximately 8% of women who have had a CS. The risk of fever, bladder injuries and surgical injuries does not vary with planned mode of birth in women who have had ≥4 Caesarean sections (*NICE*, 2011).

44. Answer E

Pelvic pain which is variable over the menstrual cycle may be hormonally-driven; for example, endometriosis. Eliciting a history of dysmenorrhoea and dyspareunia may be helpful. Moreover, association of bowel and bladder symptoms, the effect of movement and psychological factors should be considered. Sexually active women with chronic pelvic pain should be offered screening for sexually transmitted infections. Adhesions may cause pain; however, there is no evidence to support division of adhesions in women with chronic pelvic pain (*RCOG*, 2012; Green-top Guideline 41: *The initial management of chronic pelvic pain*).

45. Answer C

Shoulder dystocia is associated with previous shoulder dystocia, macrosomia, diabetes, prolonged first stage of labour, prolonged second stage of labour, oxytocin augmentation, assisted vaginal delivery and maternal body mass index >30 (*RCOG*, 2012; Green-top Guideline 42: *Shoulder dystocia*).

46. Answer E

The most common site of sepsis in the puerperium is the uterus. Clinical signs of sepsis include: fever, hypothermia, tachycardia, tachypnoea, hypoxia, hypotension, oliguria and impaired consciousness. Risk factors for sepsis include: obesity, diabetes, impaired immunity, invasive procedures, cervical cerclage, prolonged spontaneous rupture of membranes, wound haematoma and black or minority ethnic group origin (*RCOG*, 2012; Green-top Guideline 64b: *Bacterial sepsis following pregnancy*).

47. Answer B

Small-for-gestational-age (SGA) refers to an infant born with a birth weight less than the 10th centile. 50–70% of SGA fetuses may be constitutionally small. Women who have a major risk factor for SGA should be referred for serial ultrasound with umbilical artery Doppler from 26–28 weeks. Women who have three or more minor risk factors should be referred for uterine artery Doppler at 20–24 weeks of gestation (*RCOG*, 2013; Green-top Guideline 31: *The investigation and management of the small-for-gestational-age fetus*).

48. Answer A

Risk factors for placenta praevia include previous placenta praevia, previous Caesarean section, previous termination of pregnancy, multiparity, advanced maternal age, multiple pregnancy, smoking and assisted conception (*RCOG*, 2011; Green-top Guideline 63: *Antepartum haemorrhage*).

49. Answer **FTFTF**

HPV triage and test of cure has been introduced in the cervical screening programme in England. If there are borderline changes or low-grade dyskaryosis, the sample is tested for human papilloma virus (HPV). If the sample is HPV-positive, the patient is invited for colposcopy. In the case of CIN 1, if no treatment is required cytology is repeated at 12 months. If treatment is required for CIN 1, cytology is repeated at 6 months. For CIN 2/3, cytology is repeated at 6 months after treatment. Following borderline changes and negative colposcopy, routine 3- or 5-year recall is resumed (*HPV triage and test of cure*, available at www.cancerscreening.nhs.uk/cervical/hpv-triage-test-of-cure.html [last accessed 5 September 2013]).

50. Answer **TTFTF**

Small-for-gestational-age (SGA) is defined as an estimated fetal weight or abdominal circumference less than the 10th centile. If severe SGA is identified at the 18–20 week scan, a referral to a fetal medicine specialist should be offered. Karyotyping should be offered in severely SGA fetuses particularly if structural anomalies are present. Serological screening for congenital cytomegalovirus (CMV) and toxoplasmosis infection should also be offered in severe SGA. Testing for syphilis and malaria should be considered in high risk populations (*RCOG*, 2013; Green-top Guideline 31: *The investigation and management of the small-for-gestational-age fetus*).

51. Answer **TTTTT**

Risk factors for placental abruption include: pre-eclampsia, fetal growth restriction, polyhydramnios, advanced maternal age, multiparity, low body mass index (BMI), pregnancy following assisted reproductive techniques, intrauterine infection, premature rupture of membranes, abdominal trauma and smoking, as well as cocaine and amphetamine use during pregnancy (*RCOG*, 2011; Green-top Guideline 63: *Antepartum haemorrhage*).

52. Answer **TFFTT**

Functional or simple ovarian cysts which are <5 cm diameter usually resolve over 2–3 menstrual cycles. Women with simple ovarian cysts of 5–7 cm in diameter should have yearly ultrasound follow-up and those with larger simple cysts should be considered for either further imaging (MRI) or surgical intervention. A serum Ca-125 does not need to be undertaken in all premenopausal women when a simple ovarian cyst has been diagnosed on ultrasound. Lactate dehydrogenase (LDH), AFP and hCG should be measured in all women under age 40 with a complex ovarian mass, due to the risk of germ cell tumours (*RCOG/BSGE*, 2011; Joint Guideline 62: *Management of suspected ovarian masses in premenopausal women*).

53. Answer **FFFTT**

Routine screening of all pregnant women for antenatal group B streptococcus (GBS) carriage is not recommended. Antenatal prophylaxis with oral benzylpenicillin for vaginal / rectal colonisation does not reduce the risk of GBS colonisation at delivery. Intrapartum antibiotic prophylaxis should be offered to women with GBS bacteriuria. Intrapartum antibiotic prophylaxis should be offered to women who are pyrexial in labour (>38°C). For women who have accepted antibiotic therapy, benzylpenicillin should be administered after the onset of labour and given regularly until delivery. Clindamycin may be used in those who are penicillin-allergic (*RCOG*, 2012; Green-top Guideline 36: *The prevention of early-onset neonatal group B streptococcal disease*).

54. Answer **TFTTT**

Subcutaneous depot medroxyprogesterone acetate is bioequivalent to intramuscular depot medroxyprogesterone acetate (150 mg Depo-Provera). This method of contraception prevents ovulation. Both these methods may be associated with loss of bone mineral density, amenorrhoea, weight gain and a delayed return to fertility. Advantages of subcutaneous administration include the potential for self-administration; however, this is outside product licence.

55. Answer **TFFFT**

Its mode of action is primarily on ovulation inhibition by suppression of gonadotrophins, as is the case with other combined hormonal contraceptives. Current evidence suggests that Zoely has fewer effects on lipid and glucose metabolism when compared to other combined oral contraceptives. A white active tablet is taken for 24 days and an inactive yellow one for 4 days, that is, there is a 24/4 regimen with no pill-free interval. 7 days of active (white) tablets are needed to maintain ovulation suppression. Zoely may be taken continuously, i.e. missing out the inactive pills to delay withdrawal bleeding; however, the risk of breakthrough bleeding then increases.

56. Answer **FTTFT**

The additional risk of miscarriage following amniocentesis is approximately 1%. Amniocentesis should be performed after 15 weeks of gestation. Amniocentesis before 14 weeks of gestation (early amniocentesis) has a higher miscarriage rate and an increased risk of fetal talipes and respiratory morbidity. Women should be advised that the additional risk of miscarriage following chorionic villus sampling (CVS) may be slightly higher than that of amniocentesis carried out after 15 weeks of gestation. CVS should not be performed before 10 completed weeks of gestation. CVS is usually performed between 11 and 13 weeks of gestation.

57. Answer **TTFTT**

Women with lichen sclerosus and erosive lichen planus are at increased risk of a personal or family history of autoimmune disorders. Skin biopsy is not necessary when a diagnosis can be made on clinical examination. Biopsy is required if the woman fails to respond to treatment or there is clinical suspicion of VIN or cancer. Women with vulval skin disorders require examination of other mucosal sites (*RCOG*, 2011; Green-top Guideline 58: *The management of vulval skin disorders*).

58. Answer **TFTTF**

Women between 24 and 34^{+6} weeks of gestation who are at risk of preterm birth should be offered a single course of antenatal corticosteroids. Women between 23 and 23^{+6} weeks of gestation who are at risk of preterm birth should be considered for a single course of antenatal corticosteroids. Women with multiple pregnancy at risk of iatrogenic or spontaneous preterm delivery between 24^{+0} and 34^{+6} weeks of gestation should be offered antenatal steroids. Elective Caesarean section should normally be performed at or after 39 weeks of gestation to reduce respiratory morbidity. If Caesarean section is planned before this corticosteroids should be given (*RCOG*, 2010; Green-top Guideline 7: *Antenatal corticosteroids to reduce neonatal morbidity and mortality*).

59. Answer **FTFTF**

If appropriate, women should be advised to consider taking non-steroidal anti-inflammatory drugs (NSAIDs) approximately 1 hour before their outpatient hysteroscopy to reduce post-operative pain. Topical local anaesthesia should be considered if a cervical tenaculum is to be used. Local anaesthesia in the cervical canal does not reduce pain during diagnostic outpatient hysteroscopy but may reduce the incidence of vasovagal reactions. Conscious sedation should not be routinely used in outpatient hysteroscopic procedures (*RCOG*, 2011; Green-top Guideline 59: *Best practice in outpatient hysteroscopy*).

60. Answer **FFTTF**

Smoking during pregnancy increases the risk of pregnancy complications, premature delivery, intra-uterine growth restriction, stillbirth and sudden infant death syndrome. Infants of parents who smoke are more likely to suffer from serious respiratory infections, asthma and glue ear.

61. Answer **TTTTT**

Amniotic fluid embolism may occur during labour, after abdominal trauma, termination of pregnancy, placental abruption and Caesarean section. Risk factors include multiparity, advanced maternal age and trauma. It may present with acute shortness of breath and hypotension. It may be followed by cardiac arrest and disseminated intravascular coagulation.

62. Answer **FTFFT**

Echogenic bowel refers to bright loops of fetal bowel seen on the 18–20 week fetal anomaly scan. Most fetuses identified with echogenic bowel are normal; it is seen in <1% of pregnancies. It may be associated with cystic fibrosis, inflammation of the bowel serosa secondary to a congenital viral infection such as cytomegalovirus, bowel obstruction, chromosome anomalies such as trisomy 21 and intrauterine growth restriction.

63. Answer **TFTFF**

Club-foot can be classified as congenital, syndromic, or positional. It may be associated with oligohydramnios and uterine anomalies. Male fetuses are predominantly affected. The birth prevalence varies among different ethnic groups; the lowest rates are seen in Asian populations.

64. Answer **FTTFF**

PKU is an autosomal recessive condition that is part of the newborn blood spot programme. Those with PKU are unable to break down phenylalanine into tyrosine as the liver does not produce enough phenylalanine hydroxylase. A baby with untreated phenylketonuria may show developmental delay by 6 months.

65. Answer **FTFFT**

Pregnant women are at increased risk for UTIs, particularly in the 2nd trimester. The increased risk may be related to ureteral dilatation, decreased ureteral tone, increased bladder volume and decreased bladder tone. Up to 70% of pregnant women develop glycosuria, which may encourage bacterial growth in the urine.

66. Answer **FFTFF**

By the third trimester cardiac output increases by up to 50%. Stroke volume increases by 35%. Peripheral vascular resistance falls due to vasodilatation in pregnancy. There is a resultant increase in heart rate by up to 25%. Cardiac contractility remains unchanged. During pregnancy the diaphragm is displaced upwards; this results in the cardiac apex being more leftward and anterior.

67. Answer **TTFFT**

As pregnancy progresses the gravid uterus compresses the inferior vena cava and the lower aorta in the supine position. This in turn impedes venous return to the heart and therefore causes a fall in cardiac output. Aortic compression may reduce uteroplacental and renal blood flow. Left lateral tilt during Caesarean section minimises this.

68. Answer **FTTTT**

The hypothalamus secretes gonadotrophin-releasing hormone (GnRH), which stimulates the anterior pituitary gland to release follicle-stimulating hormone (FSH). This causes an ovarian dominant follicle to grow. Mid-cycle there is a surge of luteinising hormone (LH) which occurs with an FSH surge; this results in ovulation. The developing dominant follicle produces oestrogen, which stimulates endometrial proliferation. FSH and LH levels decrease when the ovum is released, corpus luteum develops at the site of the ruptured follicle, and progesterone is produced. Menstruation results from endometrial shedding due to the rapid decline in oestrogen and progesterone levels from the involuting corpus luteum, 14 days after ovulation.

69. Answer **FFFFT**

Tranexamic acid is an antifibrinolytic which is a potent competitive inhibitor of the activation of plasminogen to plasmin. Tranexamic acid may be used to treat menorrhagia. Treatment with tranexamic acid should not be initiated until menstrual bleeding has started. Contraindications include active thromboembolic disease or a history of venous or arterial thrombosis.

70. Answer **FTTTT**

Risk factors for ovarian cancer include: nulliparity, family history, BRCA1 and BRCA2 gene mutations, hereditary non-polyposis colorectal cancer.

71. Answer **TFFFT**

Women who have a BRCA1 gene mutation have a 60–90% lifetime risk of breast cancer and women who have a BRCA2 gene mutation have a 45–85% lifetime risk cancer. There is a 4–5% risk of ovarian cancer if a close relative is affected. Women with BRCA1 gene mutation have a 40–60% lifetime risk of developing ovarian cancer. Women with BRCA2 gene mutation have a 10–30% lifetime risk of developing ovarian cancer. The risk of developing ovarian cancer starts to increase from the age of 40 for BRCA1 carriers and in the mid 40s for BRCA2 carriers.

72. Answer **FTTFF**

Parvovirus B19 may cause a mild illness in a pregnant woman but infection via transplacental spread in the first 20 weeks of pregnancy can lead to intrauterine death, fetal anaemia and hydrops fetalis. Up to one-third of women are seronegative for parvovirus B19 and are therefore susceptible to infection. There is no licensed vaccine or screening programme for parvovirus B19.

73. Answer **TTTTT**

Persistent abdominal distension, symptoms suggestive of irritable bowel syndrome, satiety, pelvic or abdominal pain and increased urinary urgency and/or frequency may be associated with ovarian cancer (*NICE*, 2011; *Ovarian cancer – quick reference guide*).

74. Answer **FTTFT**

The uterine body and cervix are supplied by branches of the uterine artery, a branch of the internal iliac artery. The ovary is supplied by the ovarian artery which is a direct branch from the abdominal aorta. The right ovarian vein terminates in the inferior vena cava and the left usually drains into the renal vein. The ovary is often located in the ovarian fossa, on the lateral pelvic wall between the external and internal iliac vessels.

75. Answer **FTFTT**

Most of the lymph from the pelvis drains into nodes adjacent to the internal iliac artery; this then passes to the common iliac nodes. Lymphatic vessels from the ovaries and the rectum pass directly to the aortic nodes. Some vessels from the body of the uterus drain into the superficial inguinal nodes.

76. Answer **TFFFF**

To minimise risks to the fetus a woman would ideally stop smoking without using nicotine replacement therapy. However, the risk from continued smoking to the fetus is likely to be greater than any potential risks of nicotine replacement therapy, because there is a higher exposure to nicotine in addition to other toxins. Nicotine exposure in breast milk is minimal. Pregnant and breastfeeding women who are using nicotine patches to aid smoking cessation should be advised to remove them before going to bed. Bupropion and varenicline are not recommended for use in women who are pregnant or breastfeeding (*NICE*, 2010; *Quitting smoking in pregnancy and following childbirth* – quick reference guide PH26).

77. Answer **TFFTT**

Approximately 4–10% of women with anogenital lichen sclerosus will have steroid-resistant disease. Steroid-resistant disease may be managed with topical tacrolimus under the supervision of a specialist clinic. Women with VIN need to be seen on a regular basis for vulvoscopy; moreover, women who have been treated for VIN are at risk of intraepithelial neoplasia at other sites. The gold standard for the treatment of VIN is local surgical excision.

78. Answer **TTTTT**

Zoladex may be used in the management of endometriosis; it is usually given with add-back hormone replacement therapy to reduce bone mineral density loss and vasomotor symptoms. It is indicated for the pre-thinning of the endometrium prior to endometrial ablation or resection. It may be used in anaemic patients due to undergo surgery for fibroids.

79. Answer **TFTTT**

The *Diagnostic and Statistical Manual of Mental Disorders* (DSM IV) defines vaginismus as occurring when there is recurrent or persistent involuntary spasm of the musculature of the outer third of the vagina that interferes with intercourse and causes distress. The ability to use tampons should be elicited in the history. Physical causes of pain may include genital tract infections, vestibulitis and atrophic tissues post-menopause. Psychological associations include sexual assault and traumatic sexual experience. Management includes cognitive behavioural therapy, psychosexual therapy and the use of graded vaginal trainers.

80. Answer **FFTFF**

There have been concerns raised about the potential effects of Depo-Provera on bone mineral density (BMD), particularly in those less than 18 years and in women approaching the menopause. It is recommended that for women with significant lifestyle and/or medical risk factors for osteoporosis, other methods of contraception should be considered. Women should be informed that Depo-Provera is associated with a small loss of BMD, which is usually recovered after discontinuation. Women should be advised that there is no available evidence on the effect on long-term fracture risk. The Department of Health Medicines and Healthcare products Regulatory Agency (MHRA) advises that women on Depo-Provera are assessed on a 2-yearly basis; however, it does not advise what form the 2 year re-evaluation should take and there is no suggestion that re-evaluation includes bone density measurement.

81. Answer **TFTTF**

The ovaries are suspended with the posterior surfaces of the broad ligaments. The ovaries are attached to this by the mesovarium. However, most of the ovarian surface is devoid of peritoneum. The ovary lies in the ovarian fossa, between the external and internal iliac vessels. The ureter descends in the posterior boundary of the ovarian fossa. The ovarian artery is a direct branch from the aorta.

82. Answer **FTFFT**

Hereditary non-polyposis colorectal cancer (HNPCC) is an autosomal dominant disorder that is caused by a germline mutation in one of several DNA mismatch repair genes. This may be a causative factor in 2–3% of colorectal malignancies and 2% of endometrial cancers. It may also increase the risk of ovarian, upper urologic tract, gastric and biliary / pancreatic cancers. Women with HNPCC may have an up to 70% risk of endometrial cancer.

83. Answer **FFTTT**

Risk factors for endometrial cancer include obesity, nulliparity, late menopause, unopposed oestrogen therapy, polycystic ovarian disease, breast cancer and family history of endometrial cancer. Women who have hereditary non-polyposis colorectal cancer (HNPCC) appear to have a markedly increased risk for developing endometrial cancer.

84. Answer **TFTFT**

During pregnancy the increased blood volume and cardiac output in turn increases renal plasma flow and glomerular filtration rate (GFR). This increases urea and creatinine clearance so that plasma levels are lower than in the non-pregnant population. Plasma osmolality decreases due to water retention. Mild glycosuria and/or proteinuria can occur in normal pregnancy because the increase in GFR may exceed the renal tubules' ability for reabsorption.

85. Answer **FFTTF**

Blood volume increases from 6–8 weeks of gestation and reaches a maximum at approximately 32–34 weeks. Blood volume returns to normal 10–14 days postpartum. Plasma volume increases by 45%; however, red cell mass increases by 20–30%, resulting in haemodilution. Total body water increases secondary to renal sodium retention. The white cell count increases during pregnancy and peaks after delivery. Platelet production increases but the platelet count falls, partly due to dilution.

86. Answer **TFTTT**

Pruritus in obstetric cholestasis usually involves the palms and soles of the feet; it is usually worse at night. There is an increased risk of meconium passage, stillbirth and iatrogenic premature birth in obstetric cholestasis.

87. Answer **TTTTT**

Antenatal steroids are associated with a reduction in neonatal death rate, respiratory distress syndrome and intraventricular haemorrhage. Antenatal corticosteroids have no known benefits for the mother. Antenatal corticosteroids should be given to women for whom an elective Caesarean section is planned prior to 39 weeks of gestation.

88. Answer **TFTFT**

Women presenting with vulval dermatitis should be assessed for symptoms of urinary and/or faecal incontinence. The history should include details of any personal or family history of atopic conditions. Serum ferritin should be checked in women with vulval dermatitis. Skin patch testing should be performed for women seen with vulval dermatitis.